KU-544-138

Simpson's Forensic Medicine

Twelfth Edition

Richard Shepherd

Senior Lecturer in Forensic Medicine
Forensic Medicine Unit
St George's Medical and Dental School
Tooting, London, UK

ARNOLD

A member of the Hodder Headline Group
LONDON

First published in Great Britain in 1947
Twelfth edition published in 2003 by
Arnold, a member of the Hodder Headline Group,
338 Euston Road, London NW1 3BH

http://www.arnoldpublishers.com

Distributed in the United States of America by
Oxford University Press Inc.,
198 Madison Avenue, New York, NY10016
Oxford is a registered trademark of Oxford University Press

© 2003 Arnold

All rights reserved. No part of this publication may be
reproduced or transmitted in any form or by any means,
electronically or mechanically, including photocopying,
recording or any information storage or retrieval system,
without either prior permission in writing from the
publisher or a licence permitting restricted copying.
In the United Kingdom such licences are issued by the
Copyright Licensing Agency: 90 Tottenham Court Road,
London W1T 4LP.

Whilst the advice and information in this book are
believed to be true and accurate at the date of going to
press, neither the authors nor the publisher can accept any
legal responsibility or liability for any errors or omissions
that may be made. In particular (but without limiting the
generality of the preceding disclaimer) every effort has been
made to check drug dosages; however it is still possible that
errors have been missed. Furthermore, dosage schedules are
constantly being revised and new side-effects recognized.
For these reasons the reader is strongly urged to consult the
drug companies' printed instructions before administering
any of the drugs recommended in this book.

British Library Cataloguing in Publication Data
A catalogue record for this book is available from the
British Library

Library of Congress Cataloging-in-Publication Data
A catalog record for this book is available from the
Library of Congress

ISBN 0 340 76422 8

ISBN 0 340 81059 9 (International Students' Edition –
restricted territorial availability)

1 2 3 4 5 6 7 8 9 10

Commissioning Editor: Serena Bureau
Development Editor: Layla Vandenbergh
Project Editor: James Rabson
Production Controller: Deborah Smith
Cover Design: Stewart Larking

Typeset in 9.5/12 pt Minion by Charon Tec Pvt. Ltd,
Chennai, India

Printed and bound in India

What do you think about this book? Or any other Arnold title?
Please send your comments to feedback.arnold@hodder.co.uk

returned on or before

Simpson's
Forensic Medicine

WITHDRAWN

LIVERPOOL
JOHN MOORES UNIVERSITY
AVRIL ROBARTS LRC
TITHEBARN STREET
LIVERPOOL L2 2ER
TEL. 0151 231 4022

LIVERPOOL JMU LIBRARY

3 1111 01056 9521

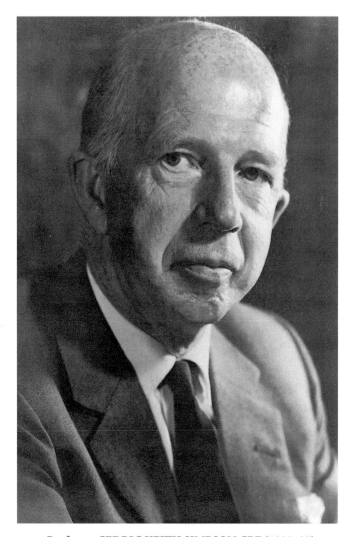

Professor CEDRIC KEITH SIMPSON CBE (1907–85)
MD (Lond), FRCP, FRCPath, MD (Gent), MA (Oxon), LLD (Edin),
DMJ

Keith Simpson was the first Professor of Forensic Medicine in the University of London and undoubtedly one of the most eminent forensic pathologists of the twentieth century. He spent all his professional life at Guy's Hospital and his name became a 'household word' through his involvement in innumerable notorious murder trials in Britain and overseas. He was made a Commander of the British Empire in 1975.

He was a superb teacher, through both the spoken and the printed word. The first edition of this book appeared in 1947 and in 1958 won the Swiney Prize of the Royal Society of Arts for being the best work on medical jurisprudence to appear in the preceding ten years.

Contents

Preface

The increasing interest in Forensic Medicine throughout the world is no doubt a result of the global rise in both crime and litigation. The advancement of the academic as well as the popular aspects of the subject have led to the continuing success of *Simpson's Forensic Medicine*.

The causes and effects of homicides, suicides and accidents and the abuse of drugs and poisons are broadly the same wherever a Forensic Practitioner works. While no single textbook can be expected to record and report all of the possible legal permutations, it is hoped that this twelfth edition of *Simpson's Forensic Medicine*, written from a broad perspective but with a firm attachment to British and European law, will serve as a useful basis for Forensic Practitioners working within any legal system. To this end, the book has been completely re-written, and new photographs and diagrams have been included to elucidate and expand the text, and, particularly, to clarify significant forensic points.

Improved techniques for the examination of both the living and the dead are continually being developed, often in response to particular events, and they are commonly associated with major advances in the Forensic Sciences. As a result, some aspects of Forensic Medicine originally described by Keith Simpson in the early editions of this textbook are now outdated. Two examples are toxicology and human identification, both of which have developed into specialities in their own right.

Toxicology has become something of a 'black box' science to Forensic Practitioners: they do not need to know the minutiae of the analytical processes. However, they do still need to know some of the fundamentals that underpin them, they must understand the effects of natural or man-made drugs and poisons,

and they must be able to interpret accurately the results provided by the toxicologist. In the field of human identification, DNA technology has all but obliterated the study of serology that was so important to Keith Simpson and his contemporaries.

As our own specialist knowledge develops and progresses we must also ensure that our basic skills continue to be reviewed and that advances in our speciality are debated, tested and validated by our forensic peers before they are presented to the courts as reliable evidence. We must never allow 'good enough' to be acceptable, since we are dealing not only with the lives of the injured or killed, and but also with the lives and the freedom of the accused. A Forensic Practitioner who lacks knowledge, skill or impartiality has no role whatsoever in today's local, national or international practice of Forensic Medicine.

Other professionals in the legal systems – the police, the lawyers and the forensic scientists – need an understanding of our skills and the limits of our knowledge so that together we can strive to improve the quality of our advice and the standard of the evidence we give to the courts. *Simpson's* has been popular with students, doctors, scientists, police officers and lawyers for many years and, it would seem, has furthered that understanding of the role of the Forensic Practitioner. It is hoped that this edition will continue that long tradition.

Whatever the future of Forensic Medicine and Science, the author's aim is that *Simpson's Forensic Medicine* will continue to provide a firm foundation for all those requiring accurate and clear information, whether in the field, the laboratory or the courtroom.

Richard Shepherd

Acknowledgements

I would like to thank my family and friends who may have noticed a degree of introspection and preoccupation during the inception, development and delivery of this book.

I would like to thank Professor Keith Simpson, as it was the third edition of this textbook, shown to me while still at school, that inspired my own interest and subsequent career in Forensic Medicine. I hope that this edition will inspire others in turn.

Author's Note

Throughout this book, the words 'he' and 'she' are used at random and where words denoting the gender are encountered, the opposite sex is equally applicable, except where the context makes it obviously inappropriate.

The Doctor and the Law

Most countries in the world have established rules and codes that govern the behaviour of the population within that country. By and large, the rules have been established over many hundreds of years and are generally accepted because they are for the mutual benefit of the population – they are the framework which prevents anarchy. Whereas there are some fundamental rules (for instance concerning the casual taking of life) that are to be found in every country, there are also considerable variations from country to country in many of the other codes or rules. The laws of a country are usually established by an elected political institution, the population accepts them and they are enforced by the imposition of penalties on those who are found guilty of breaking them.

Members of the medical profession are bound by the same general laws as the population as a whole, but they are also bound by additional laws specific to the practice of medicine. The training, qualification and registration of doctors, the use of drugs and medicines, the registration of births and deaths, and the organization of the health service may all be regarded as parts of more general medical legislation, and individual laws may be passed to deal with specific issues such as abortion, transplantation, *in-vitro* fertilization etc.

There was a time when the practice of medicine was more paternalistic and a relatively low level of legal awareness was probably acceptable. However, the increasingly litigious nature of current medical practice, especially in the Western world, suggests that it is essential for doctors to be aware of the specific laws relating to medicine.

The great diversity of the legal systems around the world poses a number of problems to the author when giving details of the law in a book such as this. Laws on the same aspect commonly differ widely from country to country, and some medical procedures (e.g. abortion) that are considered standard practice in some countries are considered to be a crime in others. Even within the British Isles, there are three main legal systems with considerable medico-legal variations: England and Wales, Scotland, and Northern Ireland. There are also smaller jurisdictions with their own individual variations in the Isle of Man and the Channel Isles. Over all of these areas there is now European legislation and with it the possibility of final appeals to the European Court. While accepting the variations between continents and countries, this book will try to present best current practice as viewed from the UK, but with the other medico-legal areas in mind.

It is important also to establish the difference between legal and ethical responsibilities. Ethical responsibilities are discussed in greater detail in Chapter 2, but, put simply, ethics are a self-imposed code of the national or international medical community which are not fixed in legislation but which are assumed or adopted voluntarily by the medical profession.

THE LEGAL SYSTEM

There are many national variations but the basic pattern is very similar. The exact structure is often rooted deep within the history or the religious beliefs of the country.

The criminal system

Criminal law deals with disputes between the state and the individual. Criminal trials involve offences that are 'against public interest'; these include offences against the person, property, public safety, security of the state etc. The dispute is between the state and the individual and in these matters the state acts as the voice or the agent of the people.

In continental Europe, a form of law derived from the Napoleonic era applies. Napoleonic law is inquisitorial and both the prosecution and the defence have to make their cases to the court, which then chooses which is the more credible. Evidence is often taken in written form as depositions, sometimes referred to as 'documentary evidence'.

The Anglo-Saxon model applies in the UK and in many, if not most, of the countries that it has influenced in the past. It is an adversarial system and so it is for the prosecution to prove their case to the jury or the magistrates 'beyond reasonable doubt'. The defence does not have to prove innocence because any individual is presumed innocent until found guilty. However, it is most unusual for the defence lawyers simply to remain silent, and they will usually attack the weaknesses of the case presented by the prosecution lawyers and also present their own evidence.

The penalties that can be imposed in the criminal system commonly include monetary charges (fines) and loss of liberty (imprisonment). Some countries allow for corporal punishment (beatings), mutilation (amputation of parts of the body) and capital punishment (execution).

Civil courts

These courts exist to resolve disputes between individuals caused by some private wrong or disadvantage that is not the concern of the state. The dispute may be based upon alleged negligence, contractual failure, debt, libel/slander etc. The state accepts that human interactions are fallible but that differences are not necessarily criminal. The civil courts can be viewed as a mechanism set up by the state that allows for the fair resolution of disputes in a structured way.

The penalty that can be imposed by these courts is designed to restore the position of the successful claimant to that which he had before the event, and is generally financial compensation (damages). In the USA there may also be a punitive part to these damages.

In both civil and criminal trials, the person against whom the action is being taken is called the defendant; the accuser in criminal trials is the state and in civil trials it is the plaintiff.

There are situations in which both types of proceeding may follow a single incident. An example is a road traffic accident following which the driver may be charged through the criminal court with traffic offences (such as dangerous driving) and sued through the civil court for the injuries he has caused to another person involved.

DOCTORS AND THE LAW

Doctors may become involved with the law in the same way as any other citizen: they may be charged with a criminal offence or they may be sued through the civil court. A doctor may also be witness to a criminal act and may be required to give evidence about it in court.

There are circumstances in which doctors become involved with the law simply because they have professional skills or experience. In these cases, the doctor may have one of two roles, which are sometimes overlapping.

Professional witness

This role is equivalent to a simple witness of an event, but occurs when the doctor is providing factual medical evidence. For instance, a casualty doctor may confirm that a leg was broken or that a laceration was present and may report on the treatment given. A general practitioner may confirm that an individual has been diagnosed as having epilepsy or angina. No comment or opinion is given and any report deals solely with medical facts.

Expert witness

An expert witness is one who expresses an opinion about medical facts. An expert will form an opinion, for instance about the cause of the fractured leg or the laceration. An expert will express an opinion about the cause of the epilepsy or the ability of an individual with angina to drive a passenger service vehicle. Before forming an opinion, an expert witness will ensure that the relevant facts about a case are made available to them and they may also wish to examine the patient.

There are often situations of overlap between these two witness roles: the dermatologist may diagnose an allergic dermatitis (professional aspect) and then comment on the role that exposure to particular chemicals may have played in the development of that dermatitis (expert aspect). Forensic pathologists will produce a report on their post-mortem examination (professional aspect) and then form conclusions based upon their findings (expert aspect).

The role of the expert in the civil courts has recently changed in the UK and the court now expects experts to report on all relevant aspects of a case and not just those aspects that are of importance to the party who has instructed them. The civil courts may now request experts from opposing sides to meet and produce a joint report. The aims of these new rules are to enable the court to identify and deal more speedily and fairly with the medical points at issue in a case.

DOCTOR IN COURT

There are many different courts in the UK: Coroner, Magistrate, Crown and the Courts of Appeal etc. Court structure in other jurisdictions will have similar complexity and, although the exact process doctors may experience when attending court will depend to some extent upon which court in which jurisdiction they attend, there are a number of general rules that can be made about giving evidence. If there is any doubt in a doctor's mind about what will happen when he attends a particular court, he should ask either the person or group (solicitor, police, state prosecution

service etc.) that is requesting him to give evidence or he can ask at the court itself.

Statement

A statement in a criminal case is a report that is prepared in a particular form so that it can be used as evidence. There is an initial declaration that ensures that the person preparing the statement is aware that he must not only tell the truth but must also ensure that there is nothing within the report that he knows to be false. The effect of this declaration is to render the individual liable for criminal prosecution if he has lied.

In civil proceedings a different official style is adopted. In these cases a sworn statement (an affidavit) is made before a lawyer who administers an oath or other formal declaration at the time of signing. This makes the document acceptable to the court.

In many countries, a statement in official form or a sworn affidavit is commonly acceptable alone and personal appearances in court are unusual. However, in the system of law based on Anglo-Saxon principles, personal appearances are common and it is the verbal evidence – tested by the defence – that is important.

If a case comes to trial, any statement made for the prosecution will be made available to all interested parties at the court; at present the same does not apply to all reports prepared for the defence in a criminal trial.

Request or order to attend court

If summoned to appear as a witness for the court, it is the duty of every citizen to comply, and attendance at court is generally presumed without the need to resort to a written order. In general, a doctor is sent a 'witness order', which is a letter informing them of the name of the accused and possibly the nature of the case, together with the time, date and place they should attend to give evidence.

In a few cases – usually when a witness has failed to attend after the usual witness order or if it is thought that a witness may be reluctant to attend the court – a formal subpoena may be issued. A subpoena is a court order signed by a judge or other court official that must be obeyed or the individual will be in contempt of court and a fine or imprisonment may result. It is rare for a doctor to be subpoened, but occasionally doctors may request such an order to demonstrate to a patient that they are unwilling to divulge the medical facts that the court is going to require them to give.

Attendance at court

Before going to court, doctors should ensure that they have all of the relevant notes, x-rays, reports etc. The notes should be organized so that the relevant parts can be easily found.

It is imperative for a witness to attend at the time stated on the witness order or subpoena, because one can never be faulted for being on time, but it is likely that witnesses will have to wait to give their evidence. Courts are usually conscious of the pressures on professional witnesses such as doctors and try hard not to keep them waiting any longer than necessary.

Giving evidence

When called into court, every witness will, almost invariably, undergo some formality to ensure that they tell the truth. This is colloquially known as 'taking the oath' or 'swearing in'. The oath may be taken using some acceptable religious text (the Bible, Koran etc.) or by making a public declaration in a standard form without the need to touch a religious artefact. This latter process is sometimes referred to as 'affirming'. However it is done, the effect of the words is the same: once the oath has been taken, the witness is liable for the penalties of perjury.

Whether a doctor is called as a witness of fact, a professional witness of fact or an expert witness, the process of giving evidence is the same. However, before describing this process it is important to remember that the doctor's overriding duty is to give evidence to assist the court.

Whoever has 'called' the witness will be the first to examine him under oath; this is called the 'examination in chief' and the witness will be asked to confirm the truth of the facts in his statement(s). This examination may take the form of one catch-all question as to whether the whole of the statement is true, or the truth of individual facts may be dealt with one at a time. If the witness is not an expert, there may be questions to ascertain how the facts were obtained and the results of any examinations or ancillary tests performed. If the witness is an expert, the questioning

may be expanded into the opinions that have been expressed and other opinions may be sought.

When this questioning is finished, the other lawyers will have the opportunity to question the witness; this is commonly called 'cross-examination'. This questioning will test the evidence that has been given and will concentrate on those parts of the evidence that are damaging to the lawyer's case. It is likely that both the facts and any opinions given will be tested.

The final part of giving evidence is the 're-examination'. Here, the original lawyer has the opportunity to clarify anything that has been raised in cross-examination but cannot introduce new topics.

The judge may ask questions at any time if he feels that by doing so he may clarify a point or clear a point of contention. However, most judges will refrain from asking questions until the end of each of the three sections noted above.

Doctor for the defence

The defence commonly needs specialist expert medical advice too. Doctors may be asked to examine living victims of crime or the accused, to consider witness statements, photographs or medical notes etc. They may also be asked to comment on 'normal' or 'standard' protocols. All of these areas have their own particular aspects and it is a foolhardy doctor who is tempted to stray outside his own area of expertise.

The initial form of advice to the solicitor acting for the defendant is a letter or a report. There may follow a conference with the solicitor or with counsel, provision of additional information and then the preparation of a final report. This is a privileged document, which does not have to be released to other parties in either a criminal or civil case. Whether or not his report is released to the court, the doctor may be requested to attend the court to listen to the evidence, in particular the medical evidence given by others. The doctor will be able to advise counsel about the questions that can be asked of the medical and other witnesses and may also be called to give evidence.

Medical reports and statements

Apart from slight differences in emphasis, there will be no essential difference between medical reports produced for legal purposes – whether for the police, the lawyers acting for the defence, an insurance company or any other instructing authority. Before agreeing to write a report, a doctor must be certain that he has the necessary training, skill and experience and, whether because of medical secrecy or confidentiality, that he is legally entitled to do so.

THE BEHAVIOUR OF A DOCTOR IN COURT

Any medico-legal report must be prepared and written with care because it will either constitute the medical evidence on that aspect of a case or it will be the basis of any oral evidence that may be given in the future. Any doctor who does not, or cannot, sustain the comments and conclusions made in the original report while giving evidence will have a difficult time during cross-examination. However, any comments or conclusions within the report are based upon a set of facts that surround that particular case. If other facts or hypotheses are suggested by the lawyers in court during their examination, a doctor should reconsider the medical evidence in the light of these new facts or hypotheses and, if necessary, should accept that, in view of the different basis, his conclusions may be different. A doctor clinging to the flotsam of his report in the face of all evidence to the contrary is as absurd as the doctor who, at the first hint of a squall, changes his view to match the direction of the wind.

Any doctor appearing before any court in either role should ensure that his or her dress and demeanour are compatible with the role of an authoritative professional. It is imperative that doctors retain a professional demeanour and give their evidence in a clear, balanced and dispassionate manner.

The oath or affirmation should be taken in a clear voice. In some courts, witnesses will be invited to sit, whereas in others they will be required to stand. Many expert witnesses prefer to stand as they feel that it adds to their professionalism, but this decision must be matter of personal preference. Whether standing or sitting, the doctor should remain alert to the proceedings and should not lounge or slouch. The doctor should look at the person asking the questions and, if there is one, at the jury when giving his answers, and should remain business-like and polite at all times.

Evidence should also be given in a clear voice that is loud enough to reach across the court room. It is extremely irritating for all those in the court who need to hear what is said if a witness has to be constantly reminded to speak up. A muttering witness also gives the impression that his evidence is not of value or that he is not comfortable with what he is saying.

When replying to questions, it is important to keep the answers to the point of the question and as short as possible: an over-talkative witness who loses the facts in a welter of words is as bad as a monosyllabic witness. Questions should be answered fully and then the witness should stop and wait for the next question. On no account should a witness try to fill the silence with an explanation or expansion of the answer. If the lawyers want an explanation or expansion of any answer, they will, no doubt, ask for it. Clear, concise and complete should be the watchwords when answering questions.

A witness, particularly a professional one, should never become hostile, angry, rude or sarcastic while giving evidence. It is important to remember that it is the lawyers who are in control in the courtroom; they will very quickly take advantage of any witness who shows such emotions. No matter how you behave as a witness, you will remain giving evidence until the court says that you are released; it is not possible to bluff, boast or bombast a way out of this situation – and every witness must remember that they are under oath. A judge will normally intervene if he feels that the questioning is unreasonable or unfair.

A witness must be alert to attempts by lawyers unreasonably to circumscribe answers: 'yes' or 'no' may be adequate for simple questions but they are simply not sufficient for most questions and, if told to answer a complex question 'with a simple "yes" or "no" doctor', they should decline to do so and, if necessary, explain to the judge that it is not possible to answer such a complex question in that way.

The old forensic adage of 'dress up, stand up, speak up, and shut up' is still applicable and it is a fool who ignores such simple advice.

PREPARATION OF MEDICAL REPORTS

The diversity of uses of a report is reflected in the individuals or groups that may request a report: the police, prosecutors, coroners, judges, medical administrators, government departments, city authorities and lawyers of all types. The most important question that doctors must ask themselves before agreeing to write a report is whether they are entitled to write such a report – they may be limited by confidentiality, medical secrecy or, of course, by lack of knowledge or expertise. The fact of a request, even from a court, does not mean that a doctor can necessarily ignore the rules of medical confidentiality; however, a direct order from a court is a different matter and should, if valid, be obeyed. If there are any doubts, contact your medical defence society or a lawyer.

Medical confidentiality is dealt with in greater detail in Chapter 2, but in general terms the consent of a living patient is required and, if at all possible, this should be given in writing to the doctor. However, in some countries the law rides roughshod over individual patients' rights and a doctor may be forced to write reports without any reference to the wishes of the patient. If no consent was provided, this should be stated in the report, as should the basis on which the report was written. In other countries, for example Belgium, the protection of medical secrecy is very strict and even the patient's written consent may not be sufficient to allow for the disclosure of medical facts by a doctor.

In most advanced, democratic countries with established civil and human rights, the police have no particular power to order a doctor to provide confidential information against the wishes of the patient, although where a serious crime has been committed the doctor has a public duty to assist the law enforcement system. It is usual for the victim of an assault to be entirely happy to give permission for the release of medical facts so that the perpetrator can be brought to justice. It is important to remember that a doctor cannot simply assume this consent, especially if the alleged perpetrator is the husband, wife or other member of the family. It is also important to remember that consent to disclose the effects of an alleged assault does not imply consent to disclose all the medical details of the victim, and a doctor must limit his report to relevant details only.

If a victim refuses to give consent or for some reason the doctor is of the opinion that he cannot make a report, there are commonly laws available to the courts to force the doctor to divulge medical information. The laws may be very specific: for instance in Northern Ireland, where terrorist shootings and explosions were common for the last quarter of the twentieth century, emergency powers make it compulsory for doctors to report any injuries due to guns or explosives. More generally, there is a duty to report some infectious diseases.

STRUCTURE OF A REPORT

The basis of most reports lies in the notes made at the time of an examination and it is important to remember that these notes may be required in court. A report should be headed with the details of the patient, including their name, date of birth and address. The doctor's address and qualifications should follow. The date of the report is clearly essential and the date(s) and place(s) of any examination(s) should be listed, as should the details of any other person who was present during the examination(s). The details of who requested the report, the reasons for requesting it and any special instructions should be documented. A brief account of the circumstances as reported to the doctor should follow. The fact of consent of the patient must be included, although the patient's signature will remain in the doctor's notes of the examination(s).

What follows next are the details of the physical examination and then the details of any treatment given. If information other than observation during a physical examination (medical records, x-rays etc.) forms part of the basis of the report, it too must be recorded. This is the end of the factual, professional report where no opinions are given. A more senior doctor or an expert in

Case no. _____   Name _____

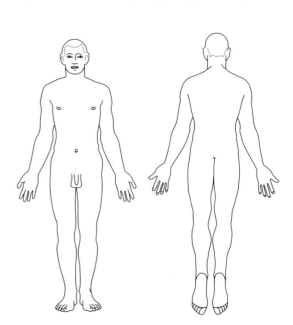

Figure 1.1 Typical body chart for marking injuries etc. in the living or the dead. A whole range of charts is available.

a particular field may well be asked to express opinions about aspects of the case and those opinions will follow the factual part of the report.

There is no great trick to writing medical reports and, to make the process simpler, they can be constructed along the same lines as the clinical notes in that they need to be structured, detailed and accurate. Do not include every single aspect of a medical history unless it is relevant. A court does not need to know every detail, but it does need to know every relevant detail, and a good report will give the relevant facts clearly, concisely and completely and in a way that an intelligent person without medical training can understand.

Medical abbreviations should be used with care and highly technical terms, especially those relating to complex pieces of equipment or techniques, should be explained in simple, but not condescending, terms. On the other hand, the courts are not medically illiterate and abbreviations in common usage such as ECG can safely be used without explanation.

It goes without saying that the contents of each and every report must be true. A report should be typed on standard-sized (A4 or foolscap) paper and not scribbled on paper torn from a drug company's advertising pad; remember it will be you who is trying to read the scribble 6 or 12 months later while under oath and under stress in the witness box. Counsel will have had weeks to decipher your writing and if even you cannot make sense of your report, it is unlikely that the court will take much notice of it. On the other hand, a clear, concise and complete report may just save you from

having to attend court at all, and if you do have to give evidence, it is so much easier to do so from a report that is legible.

Autopsy reports are a specialist type of report and may be commissioned by the coroner, the police or any other legally competent person or body. The authority to perform the examination will replace the consent given by a live patient, and is equally important. The history and background to the death will be obtained by the police or the coroner's officer, but the doctor should seek any additional details that appear to be relevant, including speaking to any clinicians involved in the care of the deceased and reviewing the hospital notes. A visit to the scene of death in non-suspicious deaths, especially if there are any unusual or unexplained aspects, is to be encouraged.

An autopsy report is confidential and should only be disclosed to the legal authority who commissioned the examination. Disclosure to others, who must be interested parties, may only be made with the specific permission of the commissioning authority and, in general terms, it would be sensible to allow that authority to deal with any requests for copies of the report.

Doctors should resist any attempt to change or delete any parts of their report by lawyers who may feel those parts are detrimental to their case; any requests to rewrite and resubmit a report with alterations for these reasons should be refused. A doctor is a witness to and for the court; he should give his evidence without fear or favour because it is for the court to decide upon the facts and not the witnesses.

The Ethics of Medical Practice

There has been a proliferation of the types of 'medical practice' that are available around the world. There is the science-based 'Western medicine', traditional Chinese medicine, Ayurvedic medicine in India, the many native systems from Africa and Asia and the rapidly proliferating modes of 'fringe medicine' in Westernized countries. These alternative forms of medicine may have their own traditions, conventions and variably active codes of conduct but we are only concerned in this book with the ethics of the science-based medical practice, 'Western medicine'.

To describe modern, science-based medicine as 'Western medicine' is historically inaccurate because its origins can be traced through ancient Greece to a synthesis of Asian, North African and European medicine. The Greek tradition of medical practice was epitomized by the Hippocratic School on the island of Cos around 400 BC. It was there that the foundations of both modern medicine and the ethical facets of the practice of that medicine were laid. A form of words universally known as the Hippocratic Oath was developed at and for those times, but the fact that it remains the basis of ethical medical behaviour, even though some of the detail is now obsolete, is a testament to its simple common sense and universal acceptance. A generally accepted translation runs as follows:

I swear by Apollo the physician and Aesculapius and Health and All-heal and all the gods and goddesses, that according to my ability and judgement, I will keep this Oath and this stipulation – to hold him who taught me this art, equally dear to me as my own parents, to make him partner in my livelihood: when he is in need of money, to share mine with him; to consider his family as my own brothers and to teach them this art, if they want to learn it, without fee or indenture. To impart precept, oral instruction and all other instruction to my own sons, the sons of my teacher and to those who have taken the disciples oath, but to no-one else. I will use treatment to help the sick according to my ability and judgement, but never with a view to injury or wrong-doing. Neither will I administer a poison to anybody when asked to do so nor will I suggest such a course. Similarly, I will not give a woman a pessary to produce abortion. But I will keep pure and holy both my life and my art. I will not use the knife, not even sufferers with the stone, but leave this to be done by men who are practitioners of this work. Into whatsoever houses I enter, I will go into them for the benefit of the sick and will abstain from every voluntary act of mischief or corruption: and further, from the seduction of females or males, of freeman or slaves. And whatever I shall see or hear in the course of my profession or not in connection with it, which ought not to be spoken of abroad, I will not divulge, reckoning that all such should be kept secret. While I carry out this oath, and not break it, may it be granted to me to enjoy life and the practice of the art, respected by all men: but if I should transgress it, may the reverse be my lot.

What is now broadly called 'medical ethics' has developed over several thousand years and is constantly being modified by changing circumstances. The laws governing the practice of medicine vary from country to country, but the broad principles of medical ethics are universal and are formulated not only by national medical associations, but by international organizations such as the World Medical Association.

Following the serious violations of medical ethics by fascist doctors in Germany and Japan during the 1939–45 war, when horrific experiments were carried out in concentration camps, the international medical community re-stated the Hippocratic Oath in a modern form in the Declaration of Geneva in 1948. This was amended by the World Medical Association in 1968 and again in 1983 and the most recent version was approved in 1994.

This declaration, made at the time of being admitted as a member of the medical profession, states that:

I solemnly pledge myself to consecrate my life to the service of humanity.

I will give to my teachers the respect and gratitude which is their due.

I will practice my profession with conscience and dignity.

The health of my patients will be my first consideration.

I will respect the secrets which are confided in me, even after the patient has died.

I will maintain by all the means in my power, the honour and noble traditions of the medical profession.

My colleagues will be my brothers and sisters.

I will not permit considerations of age, disease or disability, creed, ethnic origin, gender, nationality, political affiliation, race, sexual orientation or social standing to intervene between my duty and my patients.

I will maintain the utmost respect for human life from its beginning and even under threat I will not use my medical knowledge contrary to the laws of humanity.

I make these promises solemnly, freely and upon my honour.

INTERNATIONAL CODE OF MEDICAL ETHICS

An International Code of Medical Ethics (derived from the Declaration of Geneva) was originally adopted by the World Medical Association in 1949. The code was amended in 1968 and in 1983 and currently reads:

Duties of physicians in general

A physician shall always maintain the highest standards of professional conduct.

A physician shall not permit motives of profit to influence the free and independent exercise of professional judgement on behalf of patients.

A physician shall, in all types of medical practice, be dedicated to providing competent medical service in full technical and moral independence, with compassion and respect for human dignity.

A physician shall deal honestly with patients and colleagues and strive to expose those physicians deficient in character or competence or who engage in fraud or deception.

The following practices are deemed to be unethical conduct:

a. Self-advertising by physicians, unless permitted by the laws of the country and the Code of Ethics of the National Medical Association.
b. Paying or receiving any fee or other consideration solely to procure the referral of a patient or for prescribing or referring a patient to any source.

A physician shall respect the rights of patients, of colleagues and of other health professionals and shall safeguard patient confidences.

A physician shall act only in the patient's interest when providing medical care which might have the effect of weakening the physical and mental condition of the patient.

A physician shall use great caution in divulging discoveries or new techniques or treatment through non-professional channels.

A physician shall certify only that which he has personally verified.

Duties of physicians to the sick

A physician shall always bear in mind the obligation of preserving human life.

Table 2.1 Declarations of the World Medical Association 1970–2001

Date	Name	Subject
1970	The Declaration of Oslo	Therapeutic abortion
1973	The Declaration of Munich	Racial, political discrimination etc. in medicine
1975	The Declaration of Tokyo	Torture and other cruel and degrading treatment or punishment
1975	The Declaration of Helsinki	Human experimentation and clinical trials
1981	The Declaration of Lisbon	Rights of the patient
1983	The Declaration of Venice	Terminal illness
1983	The Declaration of Oslo	Therapeutic abortion
1984	The Declaration of San Paulo	Pollution
1987	The Declaration of Madrid	Professional autonomy and self-regulation
1987	The Declaration of Rancho Mirage	Medical education
1989	The Declaration of Hong Kong	The abuse of the elderly
1995	The Declaration of Lisbon	The rights of the patient
1996	The Declaration of Helsinki	Biomedical research involving human subjects
1997	The Declaration of Hamburg	Support for doctors refusing to participate in torture or other forms of cruel inhuman or degrading treatment
1998	The Declaration of Ottawa	The right of the child to health care

A physician shall owe his patients complete loyalty and all the resources of his science. Whenever an examination or treatment is beyond the physician's capacity, he should summon another physician who has the necessary ability.

A physician shall observe absolute confidentiality on all he knows about his patient even after the patient has died.

A physician shall give emergency care as a humanitarian duty unless he is assured that others are willing and able to give such care.

Duties of physicians to each other

A physician shall behave towards his colleagues as he would have them behave towards him.

A physician shall not entice patients from his colleagues.

A physician shall observe the principles of the Declaration of Geneva approved by the World Medical Association.

The fact that both the Declaration of Geneva and the International Code of Medical Ethics have had to be amended during the past 50 years serves to remind us that medical ethics are not static. Both the practice of medicine and the societies in which doctors work change, and medical ethics must alter to reflect these changes. The World Medical Association has adopted a number of other important declarations over the years, providing international guidance, and sometimes support, for doctors everywhere (Table 2.1).

MEDICAL ETHICS IN PRACTICE

There are many aspects of medical ethics and the subject has blossomed to the point where there are now Institutes of Medical Ethics and full-time specialists called medical ethicists.

It is hard to find any medical activity that does not have some ethical considerations, varying from research on patients to medical confidentiality, from informed consent to doctor–doctor relationships. Many older ethical considerations have progressed into law, while new concerns have arisen. But despite all this change, the basic nature of ethical behaviour remains the same and all medical ethics can be said to rest on the principle that 'The patient is the centre of the medical universe around which all the efforts of doctors revolve'.

The doctor exists for the patient, not the other way around. The doctor must never do anything to or for a patient that is not in the best interests of that patient and all other considerations are irrelevant in that doctor–patient relationship. From this one simple statement spring all other aspects of ethical behaviour, including the interaction of doctor with doctor and of doctor with society and with government.

The general principle which guides ethical behaviour is 'peer conduct', in that, even if some action is not strictly illegal in terms of the national laws, that action should not be carried out if it is against the accepted behaviour of medical colleagues. In other words, even if a doctor thinks he can 'get away with it' under the national criminal or civil laws, the disapproval of his fellow doctors – often reinforced by professional disciplinary procedures – should deter them from acting in that way.

International codes are quite clear and virtually all national medical associations subscribe to them in theory, if, regrettably, less strictly in practice. The disciplinary process and the sanctions that can be applied against the doctor found guilty of unethical practices by the General Medical Council in the UK are described in more detail in Chapter 3 and range from a public admonishment to permanent erasure from the register.

Though the spectrum of unethical conduct is wide, certain universally relevant subjects are recognized. The seriousness with which each is viewed may vary considerably in different parts of the world.

- A doctor's over-riding consideration is to the patient, while also accepting that doctors have a duty to their medical colleagues and to the community at large. The patient is the reason for the doctor's existence and all other matters must be subservient to this fact. A doctor cannot abandon his patient without ensuring that medical care is handed over to someone equally competent. A doctor cannot simply leave a patient because it is the end of his shift for that day nor can he refuse to continue long-term treatment without ensuring that some other doctor takes that person into care.
- The doctor must always do what he thinks is best for the patient's physical and mental health without consideration of race, wealth, religion, nationality etc. The doctor must act independently, or with other doctors, free of political or administrative doctrines or pressure to establish a diagnosis and to carry out treatment. However, financial resources can be limited and health 'priorities' may be dictated by administrators and politicians and so doctors may find themselves in situations where resources are limited and treatment options are denied. This may pose significant ethical dilemmas for the treating doctor.

- Doctors must act reasonably and courteously to each other for the patient's benefit as the best regimen of treatment cannot be provided by doctors split by professional or personal disputes or jealousy. A doctor should not interfere in the treatment of a patient except in an emergency when discussion with the treating doctor is not possible. If emergency treatment is provided, the patient's usual doctor should be informed as soon as possible about the nature and extent of this emergency treatment. A doctor should not criticize another doctor's judgement or treatment directly to the patient except in extreme and unusual situations, but should instead confront the other doctor directly if it is thought that the maximum benefit is not being offered to the patient. If a doctor is concerned about the professional skills or the health of a colleague, he is morally obliged to draw those concerns to the attention of the authorities.

MEDICAL CONFIDENTIALITY

Secrecy is now termed 'confidentiality', but whatever it is called it is as vital now as when the Hippocratic Oath was written. It is a fundamental tenet that whatever a doctor sees or hears in the life of his patient must be treated as totally confidential. The British Medical Association (BMA) defines confidentiality as 'the principle of keeping secure and secret from others, information given by or about an individual in the course of a professional relationship'. There are, however, exceptions to this fundamental rule, which are discussed later.

The concept of medical confidentiality is also directed at the well-being of the patient and assumes that if people cannot be confident that what they tell their doctor will stay secret, they are much less likely to reveal everything during a consultation, especially in intimate matters concerning their sex life, social and moral behaviour, use or abuse of drugs or alcohol and even their excretory functions. As a result, the clinical history may be deficient or even misleading and the best diagnosis and hence the best treatment may not be provided.

The doctor must therefore keep everything he hears to himself and it must be appreciated that the 'secrecy' belongs to the patient, not the doctor. The latter is merely the guardian of the patient's confidential matters, which does not cease on the death of the patient.

Giving health information that can be identified as belonging to a particular individual is termed 'disclosure'. Healthcare information may only be disclosed in the following situations, although different countries may have variations of this list.

- *With the consent of the patient.* If an adult patient gives consent for disclosure of information, in most countries the doctor is free so to do. The crucial feature in this process is the consent given by the patient, which is defined by the BMA as 'a decision freely made in appreciation of its consequences'. However, as already mentioned in Chapter 1, some countries have much stricter laws about the disclosure of medical information.

   An individual with 'parental responsibility' for an immature minor may consent to the disclosure of their medical information, but the situation regarding mentally incapacitated adults is slightly more complicated.

- *To other doctors.* The keeping of medical notes and records is universal, indeed a doctor would be negligent not to keep such records. These records are used to assist in the provision of health care to the patient and, in the absence of evidence to the contrary, it is assumed that patients have given 'implied consent' for the sharing of their health information on a 'need to know' basis with other healthcare professionals, who should be under the same obligation of secrecy as the doctor. However, it must be admitted that as multidisciplinary teams grow ever bigger, it is becoming increasingly difficult to control information, which now reaches an ever-widening circle of people.

- *To relatives.* In most circumstances, close relatives are told of the nature of the patient's illness, especially if they live together and have to care for the patient at home. However, this disclosure is by no means automatic and, if the patient requests that a relative is not told, the doctor must abide by that wish. If there is a medical reason why the relative should be told, this can be discussed with the patient, but the doctor cannot disclose the information in the face of refusal by the patient unless not to do so would place the relatives at risk. This dilemma is now faced, for example, when one family member has been diagnosed as having active pulmonary tuberculosis.

   Particular caution is required over the disclosure of sexual matters, such as pregnancy, abortion or venereal disease, as disclosure might cause severe conflict between close relatives such as husband and wife. In some societies the senior male relative may play a dominant role in the family and may well insist on the doctor providing him with medical information on anyone in the family, irrespective of the wishes of the individual. While remaining aware of the various ethnic and religious factors, a doctor must resist if patients themselves will not give informed consent to the release of the information. Where immature children are concerned, it is obvious that all possible information must be given to the parents or those with parental responsibility. Mature children pose different problems and, if a doctor considers them to be sufficiently mature, they may make their own decisions, which must be followed by the doctor. Such a child may also deny his parents access to his medical records.

- *Statutory (legal) requirements.* The absolute duty of medical confidentiality has, in reality, been considerably diminished. Many national laws now force the doctor to reveal what are essentially medical secrets and many are so commonplace that they are not even thought about and the whole community accepts them without question, for example official notification of births, deaths and stillbirths. In addition, statutory notification is required of many infectious diseases and occupational diseases, as are the details of therapeutic abortions, drug addiction etc. Doctors are citizens and have to obey the law of the land and so they have to submit to these regulations and patients cannot complain about their doctor revealing these types of personal information. The patient has no right of refusal, but should be notified about what information will be provided and to whom.

- *In courts of law.* Where a doctor is a witness before a court or tribunal, the magistrate, judge, coroner etc. has the power to force the doctor to disclose any relevant medical facts. The doctor may protest or ask if he can write down the confidential facts so that the public and press in court do not hear the answer. However, if the judge so directs, the doctor must answer, on pain of a fine or even imprisonment for 'contempt of court'. In such circumstances, the evidence given by the doctor is totally privileged and thus the patient cannot bring a legal action for breach of confidence.

- *The police.* In most Western countries the police have no greater power to demand the disclosure of medical information by a doctor than anyone else. There are a few well-defined circumstances, not specifically related to medical information or to medical practice, in which the police can require disclosure of information by any citizen; these involve terrorist activity and information that may identify a driver alleged to have committed a traffic offence.

The police usually require information concerning an assault on a patient, but where assault occurs within a family, such as between spouses or close relatives, the victim may not wish to bring criminal charges and so the doctor must not automatically assume that consent for disclosure will have be given.

- *Disclosure by police surgeons (forensic medical examiners).* A doctor examining a patient, usually a victim or alleged perpetrator, at the request of the police owes the same duty of confidentiality to that patient as any other doctor, and any information that is not relevant to any criminal proceedings must be given the same protection as any other medical information. The doctor in this situation may, however, disclose medical facts that are relevant to a crime, but the patient should be made aware of this before the examination begins. If ordered by a court to disclose other information gained from this examination, the doctor must, of course, comply.
- *In the public good.* This is a most difficult issue and it must be left to the doctor's own conscience whether he should reveal matters which affect people other than the patient. For instance, if a doctor learns of a serious crime (e.g. by treating wounds of an assailant that he knows must have originated in a serious assault or rape), then the issue of confidentiality clashes with the need to protect some individual or the public at large from possible further danger. The same issue may arise where a doctor suspects that a child patient is being physically or mentally abused, but here the over-riding consideration is the safety of the child.

  More commonly, the dilemma for a doctor arises from disease rather than injuries. If a serious illness in a patient poses a potential threat of 'serious harm' to the safety or health of either the patient or the public, the doctor must decide whether to break silence about the condition, for example in the case of a bus driver with serious hypertension or a teacher with tuberculosis or

some other infective disease. Usually, people in positions of public responsibility are required to disclose significant illness to their employers and to have occupational medical checks performed on behalf of the employer or licensing authority.

  The proper course is for the doctor to explain the risks to the patient and to persuade him to allow the doctor to report the problem to his employers. The patient may, of course, refuse. It is always wise to seek the advice of senior colleagues or of a professional insurance organization or national medical association before making any disclosure.
- *Disclosure to lawyers.* Lawyers have no automatic right to obtain medical information and records without the patient's consent, but in general, if a lawyer in a civil case wishes to obtain medical records and these are denied to him, he may apply to the court for 'disclosure'. In the UK the Access to Health Records Act 1990 means that this request will be granted if a lawyer can show that his client has reasonable grounds for wishing to see medical records; these grounds may be either to discover if there are grounds for a legal action or to obtain evidence for an action already commenced.

  When asked by a lawyer for a medical report, a doctor should always insist on seeing written permission for the disclosure of information signed by the individual about whom the report is to be written. If a doctor releases confidential information to another party without the consent of the patient, he may be sued or face disciplinary action by the regulatory medical authorities for unethical behaviour.

CONSENT TO MEDICAL TREATMENT

No adult person need accept medical treatment unless they wish to do so. However, if they do desire medical attention, they must give valid consent. Permission for diagnosis and treatment is essential as otherwise the doctor may be guilty of assault if he touches or even attempts to touch an unwilling person. In Britain, young persons over the age of 16 can choose their own doctor and children of this age are presumed to be competent to give permission for any treatment. Below the age of 16 there is no presumption of competency, but if the doctor thinks they are mature enough to understand, they can still give valid consent. There is no lower age limit to this competency, the crucial test being the child's ability to comprehend and to make a rational decision. Interestingly, a decision by a child under 18 to refuse treatment is not necessarily binding upon a doctor and may be overridden by those with parental responsibility or by a court.

The situation in which an adult lacks the capacity, for whatever reason, to make an informed decision is somewhat confused. Where a patient is suffering from a mental condition, and is detained in hospital under mental health legislation, he may be given treatment for his mental condition without his consent. However, the legislation does not extend to other types of medical treatment. The Adults with Incapacity Act applies in Scotland only, and allows people over 16 years to appoint a proxy decision maker to whom they delegate the power to consent to medical treatment, but only if the patient has lost the capacity to do so.

In an emergency, such as an accident where the victim is in extremis, unconscious or shocked, no permission is necessary and doctors must do as they think best for the patient in those urgent circumstances. As long as medical intervention was made in good faith for the benefit of the victim, no subsequent legal action based on lack of consent is likely to succeed.

Consent to medical treatment is of two types.

Implied consent

Most medical practice is conducted under the principle of 'implied consent', where the very fact that a person has presented at a doctor's surgery to be examined, or asks the doctor to visit him, implies that he is willing to undergo the basic clinical methods of examination, such as history taking, observation, palpation and auscultation etc. It does not extend to intimate examinations such as vaginal and rectal examinations or to invasive examinations such as venepuncture. These intimate and invasive tests should be discussed with patients and their express consent specifically obtained after explaining what is to be done and why. Refusal of consent for the procedure precludes the test or examination.

Express consent

Where complex medical procedures are concerned, more specific permission must be obtained from the patient, this being called 'express consent', and if the same procedure is repeated on another occasion, further express consent must again be obtained.

Express consent may often be obtained in writing, but this is not a legal requirement and written consent is not more valid than verbal consent. However, written consent is much easier to prove at a later date should any dispute ever arise. Ideally, either verbal or written consent should be witnessed by another person, who should also sign any document.

Consent only extends to what was explained to the patient beforehand and nothing extra should be done during the operation for which express consent has not been obtained. This can pose a dilemma for a surgeon if something unexpected is found at operation that necessitates a change of procedure.

The concept of informed consent

Consent is not legally valid unless the patient understands what he or she is giving the doctor permission to do and why the doctor wants to do it, and it may well be that the patient, having weighed up the risks, the pain and discomfort and many other factors, may decline the operation and it is their right to be able to do this. There is some room for clinical judgement and a doctor may withhold some information he believes may cause mental anguish that would adversely affect the patient's health or recovery. However, any withholding of facts may need to be justified at a later date and careful notes should be kept of any matters discussed, or specifically not discussed, during the process of obtaining express consent.

The question of consent has usually been considered by the medical and surgical teams at hospitals and as long as junior doctors conform to the protocols laid down by those teams they will not be personally responsible for any failings or omissions later discovered in the process as a whole.

Medical Malpractice

The term medical malpractice covers all failures in the conduct of doctors but only where it impinges upon their professional skills, ability and relationships. Malpractice can be conveniently divided into two broad types:

1 Medical negligence – where the standard of medical care given to a patient is considered to be inadequate.
2 Professional misconduct – where the personal, professional behaviour falls below that which is expected of a doctor.

MEDICAL NEGLIGENCE

Medical treatment is not provided with an absolute guarantee of complete success. Improvements in medical science and techniques have markedly reduced the rate of complications and unexpected outcomes from all types of treatment, but they will never disappear completely. However, all patients have the legal right to expect a satisfactory standard of medical care from their doctor even though it is accepted that this can never mean that the doctor can guarantee a satisfactory outcome to the treatment.

Most legal actions for negligence in countries with an Anglo-Saxon system of law remain within the civil law, in which a patient brings a personal action against the doctor or hospital, and to understand the concept of medical negligence certain principles must be considered.

Before a patient can succeed in a civil action for negligence against a doctor, it must be established:

1 that the doctor had a duty of care towards the patient; (and)
2 that there was a failure in that duty of care; (which)
3 resulted in physical or mental damage.

1 Once it is established that there is a duty of care, the doctor must then provide both diagnosis and treatment at a reasonable 'standard of care' – that is, consistent with the doctor's own experience and training. A junior doctor is not expected to have as much expertise as a specialist but is expected to possess at least the minimum skills tested by the qualifying examinations and, in addition, is expected to apply the level of experience consistent with his or her postgraduate training. It is accepted that doctors cannot be expected to know the details of every single recent advance in all areas of medicine, but the patient can expect a doctor to have kept up to date with major developments in his own and in closely related fields, now often referred to as Continuing Professional Development (CPD).

2 For negligence to be established, there must be a 'breach' of this standard of care, either by omission (failing to do something) or by commission (doing something wrong). It is accepted that the circumstances under which a doctor treats a patient may have a considerable bearing on the reasonable standard of care that the patient may expect; for example treatment in an acute emergency when there is neither the time nor the facilities may legitimately be less ideal than that given for the same condition in a non-urgent situation. The test of negligence that is applied relies upon the response of the average doctor with the same medical background, placed in identical circumstances.

3 Even if a patient can prove the presence of a duty of care and a breach of the standard of care, he cannot succeed in a legal action unless he can also show that he has suffered physical or mental damage. If a doctor prescribes some obviously inappropriate or even harmful medicine but the patient refuses to take the medicine, the patient cannot then recover compensation from the doctor because he has suffered no damage.

It is important to note that 'damage', in the sense of injury or harm, is quite different from 'damages', which is the financial compensation awarded to a successful litigant.

There is rarely any dispute over whether the doctor owed the patient a duty of care; the major problem is usually proof of a breach of that duty and the onus lies on the plaintiff to show that a breach occurred and not on the defendant to prove that it did not. The only exception occurs when the facts are so glaringly obvious that they need no explanation (legally *res ipsa loquiter*, or 'the facts speak for themselves'); in this situation the doctor is forced, if he can, to provide an explanation for his actions. If a patient goes into an operating theatre to have the right leg amputated and the left leg is removed instead, there is no dispute that the treatment is incorrect and the responsibility shifts to the defending doctor to explain the error.

The great problem of alleged medical negligence lies in the continuum of 'standard of care' between actions that are accepted medical practice and those that constitute a lack of care. At the junction of these two extremes is a grey area of debatable clinical judgement where some doctors would act in one way whereas others would act, quite legitimately, in a different way.

To complicate matters further, errors of clinical judgement which lead to a bad result are not always negligent. If the error results from decisions made in good faith, based on all the information that could reasonably be expected to be available at the time but which are recognized, in retrospect, to be an error, they cannot be considered to be a breach of either the duty or the standard of care.

The only way to resolve the problem of whether an act is truly negligent is by 'peer judgement', and this is the means by which most medical disputes are settled, at least in the UK. The facts of the case are placed before experts in that particular specialty and their views sought. It is sufficient in this context to show only that a substantial number of doctors agree with the actions of the defendant; there is no need for unanimity of either condemnation or support.

Most allegations of medical negligence never come before a court of law for decision. Some cases cannot be defended as far as the doctor is concerned and these will be settled by financial negotiation, either directly or, more commonly, through the medical insurers, without further argument. Other cases cannot be substantiated by the plaintiff and are eventually abandoned, often on legal advice. Of the remainder, less than half go through the full process of investigation in which each 'side' obtains expert opinions from independent medical specialists. The strength of these opinions is then reviewed and often the experts and lawyers meet to try to reach common ground and a settlement, and only if there is a wide gap between the expert opinions is the case likely to go to court for a judge to decide on the relative merits of each argument. Recent changes in the process of civil litigation in the UK have resulted in greater collaboration between the experts who, amongst other things, now have to state clearly in their reports that they understand that their primary duty is to the court and not to the party who instructs them; this has greatly reduced, if not prevented entirely, the 'hired gun' expert.

There is a common legal principle in employment that 'the master is responsible for the acts of his servants' and this principle applies to all of the employees – technicians, nurses etc. as well as to the medical staff – and so hospitals are now responsible for the actions of their staff. The cost of assuming these risks has to be met out of annual health budgets and so the continued escalation of negligence actions has resulted in a significant, and increasing, cost to the employers. It is very important to emphasize that medical insurance provided by an employing hospital or health authority does not extend to any work outside that establishment and all private specialists, general practitioners and all doctors undertaking emergency, locum or casual work continue to need personal insurance for their practice of medicine.

In many countries, commercial insurance companies provide indemnity for doctors, but other countries have mutual non-profit schemes, often run by the medical profession. These mutual insurance organizations will often take a more robust view of their members' interest and professional standing and are less likely to settle a case simply for the sake of financial expediency than either commercial firms or an employing health authority.

SYSTEMS OF COMPENSATION

The situation described above is the 'fault' system, whereby the patient has to prove that the doctor was in breach of a duty of care before he can get a single penny in damages. The system relies upon the lower level of proof available in law – the balance of probability. As a result, it is an 'all or nothing' system, for if the balance of probability of fault is assessed at 51 per cent, the patient may get a large award of damages, whereas in the same case, if the probability of fault is only 49 per cent, he gets nothing at all.

In addition, the legal process can be very slow and it will often take a number of years to settle quite a simple claim. A recent change in the law regarding the payment of lawyers now means that they can work for an agreed percentage of the damages their clients receive if they are successful; the balance to that method of payment is that they will have worked for nothing if the case does not succeed. This simple idea has been clouded by the interposition of a number of complex insurance schemes and possible litigants should study very carefully the terms and conditions of any contract that they sign to get 'free' legal assistance for a civil medical claim.

It is a socially illogical and wholly unjust situation that a patient injured by an act deemed by a court to be negligent will receive damages, whereas another patient with the same injuries resulting from an act that is not deemed negligent will receive nothing. Some countries, such as Sweden, Finland, Norway and New Zealand, with high levels of state-funded social security have introduced 'no-fault' systems whereby the test for compensation is not the presence or absence of the doctor's negligence, but rather the patient's needs. This concept is by no means new in

non-medical fields; in Britain, industrial injuries compensation has been in existence for over 40 years, the requisite funding coming from employers, employees and the state, and compensation for injuries due to criminal acts has been paid entirely by the state through the Criminal Injuries Compensation Authority for over a decade.

COMPENSATION AND DAMAGES

If a plaintiff is successful, either in a court action or by settlement between the lawyers for the parties out of court, damages will be paid. The object of this award of money is to try to restore the patient to the financial state that he was in before the incident and in addition there may be additional sums to compensate for pain, suffering and loss of quality of life. If the individual is not able to continue with his chosen work, a large part of any damages will relate to this loss of earnings, and the amount paid will clearly depend upon the nature of the work and the remuneration that the individual had been receiving or might reasonably be expected to receive.

Other damages may be based on the need for long-term nursing and special care in the future. A brain-damaged child or young person may require 24-hour attention for the rest of his life, which accounts for the huge damages awarded to infant victims of cerebral hypoxia. Similarly, the costs of future treatment to remedy some negligent damage may be calculated, though where free state medicine is available, the money will be correspondingly reduced. Pain, suffering and loss or reduction in the quality of life are usually compensated on a modest scale.

Where death has been caused, the dependent relatives (if there are any) will receive compensation for the loss of salary of the family breadwinner. The death of a child is poorly compensated as it can have no dependants and no forecast as to its level of future earnings can be made.

TYPES OF MEDICAL NEGLIGENCE

It is impossible to give a complete list of negligent situations in medical practice. An English judge once stated that 'the categories of negligence are never closed', which must be correct as every new technique that is developed provides more opportunity for something

LIVERPOOL JOHN MOORES UNIVERSITY
LEARNING SERVICES

to go wrong. However, there is a central core of situations that frequently give rise to allegations of negligence.

Obstetrics and gynaecology

- Brain damage in the newborn due to hypoxia from prolonged labour: these cases form some of the most expensive claims, currently often well in excess of several million pounds sterling. It has been suggested that fear of litigation for this has resulted in an unacceptably high rate of caesarian births.
- Failed sterilization by tubal surgery resulting in unwanted pregnancy.
- Complications of hysterectomy, such as ureteric ligation and vesicovaginal fistulae.

Orthopaedics and accident surgery

- Missed fractures, especially of the scaphoid, skull, femoral neck and cervical spine.
- Tissue and nerve damage from over-tight plaster casts.
- Undiagnosed intracranial haemorrhage.
- Missed foreign bodies in eyes and wounds, especially glass.
- Inadequately treated hand injuries, especially tendons.

General surgery

- Delayed diagnosis of acute abdominal lesions.
- Retention of instruments and swabs in operation sites.
- Operating on the wrong patient.
- Operating on the wrong limb, digit or even organ.
- Operating on the wrong side of the body.
- Failed vasectomy, without warning of lack of total certainty of subsequent sterility.
- Diathermy burns.

General medical practice

- Failure to visit a patient on request, with consequent damage.
- Failure to diagnose myocardial infarcts or other medical conditions.

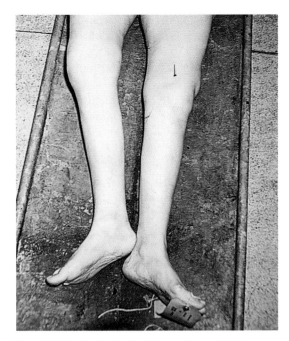

Figure 3.1 This classical fractured hip was diagnosed in the mortuary after the patient had been in hospital for a number of days with a minor head injury, but no one had examined her legs.

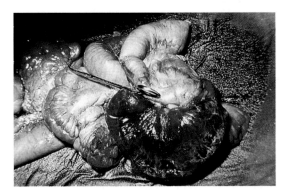

Figure 3.2 Artery forceps negligently left in the abdomen during an operation caused fatal intestinal obstruction 6 weeks later.

- Failure to refer a patient to hospital or for specialist opinion.
- Toxic results of drug administration.

Anaesthesiology

- Hypoxia resulting in brain damage.
- Neurological damage from spinal or epidural injections.

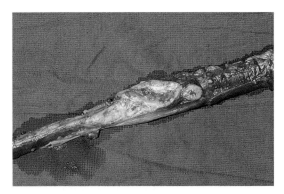

Figure 3.3 Necrosis of the spinal cord following excessive intrathecal injection of penicillin. Thirty times the proper dose was given, due to misreading the label on the box.

- Peripheral nerve damage from splinting during infusion.
- Incompatible blood transfusion.
- Incorrect or excessive anaesthetic agents.
- Allowing awareness of pain during anaesthesia.

General errors

- Failure to act on radiological or laboratory reports.
- Inadequate clinical records and failure to communicate with other doctors involved in the treatment of a patient.
- Failure to admit to hospital when necessary.
- Failure to obtain informed consent to any procedure.
- Administration of incorrect type or quantity of drugs, especially by injection.

In general, all doctors need to be constantly aware of the risks of their professional duties but not so obsessed with the possibility of legal consequences that they avoid using a potentially risky treatment that may offer considerable benefit to the patient. The practice of 'defensive medicine' may lead to the withholding of beneficial treatment to the majority because of a statistical risk to the minority.

PROFESSIONAL MISCONDUCT

The professional behaviour of a doctor, either in connection with his treatment of patients or in other areas of his behaviour, may lead to allegations of misconduct that are separate from the civil actions for negligence discussed in the previous section. Where the personal or professional conduct of a doctor is seriously criticized, his worthiness to continue as a recognized member of the medical profession may be at stake. This aspect is dealt with by various tribunals of the official authority responsible in that particular country for granting registration or a licence to practise medicine. These tribunals can examine the fitness of any doctor to remain an accredited physician and this mechanism of referral and review is designed primarily to protect the public from unsuitable or even dangerous doctors.

Because national systems of licensing and registration vary so widely, it is impossible to describe any universal rules. Nevertheless, there is a general level of ethical behaviour, morality and competence that should be subscribed to by doctors all over the world. These high standards are not born of snobbery or elitism but of practical necessity, for if patients are to derive the maximum benefit from diagnosis and treatment, they must be confident that their physician is responsible, diligent, honest and discreet. It is believed that patients are less likely to reveal intimate details of their medical history or to cooperate in treatment without the necessary ingredient of faith and confidence in the treating doctor. Thus doctors must actually possess, and be seen to possess, all the better qualities that will befit them to manage life-and-death issues.

Every country has a system for admitting new doctors to a regulated list of competent practitioners; this list is usually limited to those who have passed the final examinations of a university medical school or other accrediting institution. This initial registration or licensing will allow newly qualified doctors to commence their postgraduate training with the 'house year' or internship and this will be followed by a wide range of postgraduate training schemes and qualifications. The doctor's professional career is dependent upon remaining registered or licensed until retirement or death.

Each country may have widely different criteria that define professional misconduct; some states are very strict about the behaviour of their doctors, whereas others, unfortunately, have far too lenient an attitude. The regulatory system for professional conduct also varies greatly from place to place and, in general terms, it is most organized where the criteria for professional conduct are most strict and applied with most diligence. In many countries, the regulation and licensing of doctors are organized by the government, usually through its ministry of health or equivalent; in other countries, a more independent national medical association has a similar role.

It used to be thought that the most satisfactory system is one in which doctors themselves administer the system, preferably with statutory backing from the legislature, but which has with no direct control by government administrators or bureaucrats. Such a system existed in Britain, where the supervision of doctors' ethical behaviour is probably the strictest in the world, and for a century or so it managed the control of doctors with the support of both the profession and the public. Towards the end of the last century there was considerable public disquiet at what was seen to have become a mechanism to protect doctors from complaint rather than a mechanism to protect the public from failed and failing doctors. This disquiet triggered a major review of the structure and functions of the General Medical Council (GMC).

THE GENERAL MEDICAL COUNCIL

Established on the initiative of the British Medical Association in 1858, the GMC was set up primarily to allow the public to distinguish between properly qualified doctors and the thousands of 'quacks' that existed in the nineteenth century. The GMC did this by publishing an annual list, the Medical Register. To be included in the register, a doctor had to prove that he had passed reputable medical examinations and so the GMC gained a prime interest in the standards of medical schools and their examination standards. The GMC was also given disciplinary powers by Parliament so that it could remove misbehaving doctors from the register.

At the start of this new millennium, the GMC has undergone a period of major review and it has been recommended to the government that legislation be laid before Parliament to reduce the membership of the council from 104 (a quarter of whom are lay members) to 35, of whom 19 will be elected medical members, 2 will be appointed medical members and 14 will be lay members. The GMC will continue to work through a group of committees that cover education, standards of practice, registration and professional conduct. The work of all of these committees is overseen by the GMC.

Conduct procedures

When a complaint is made to the GMC, it is initially reviewed by a medically qualified screener who will assess:

1 how serious the matter is;
2 if the GMC has any other information or complaints about the doctor involved;
3 what evidence is available about the events.

The medical screener may reach one of a number of decisions.

1 They may decide that no further action should be taken, in which case the complaint is reviewed by a lay member of the GMC and, if both agree that no further action is to be taken, the case is dropped, but if they disagree, the complaint will pass to the Preliminary Proceeding Committee (PPC).
2 They may consider that there is no evidence of serious professional misconduct but may still find that the professional performance of the doctor has been seriously deficient and refer the complaint to an Assessment Referral Committee (ARC). There are also health procedures that can be followed if the screener forms the opinion that the doctor is in need of medical assistance himself.
3 They may consider that the complaint does relate to the conduct of the doctor and may refer it to the PPC.

The PPC is also notified of all criminal convictions of doctors so that they can assess the significance of these convictions to the practice of the doctor.

The PPC may take one of four decisions:

1 to refer the case to the Professional Conduct Committee (PCC) for a public hearing;
2 to send the doctor a letter with advice or a warning about his future practice;
3 to refer the case for further investigation into the health of the doctor;
4 to take no further action.

The PCC is restricted by law to considering charges of serious professional misconduct against a doctor. The committee is chaired by a senior lawyer who can advise its members on the law. The committee holds its hearings and announces its decisions in public but its deliberations are held in private. Evidence is heard according to strict legal procedures and is presented to the committee by lawyers acting for the GMC and the doctor. Witnesses are summonsed to appear and evidence is given under oath and the witnesses are questioned by both the lawyers and the members of the committee.

After hearing the evidence, the committee must decide whether or not the doctor is guilty of 'serious professional misconduct'. The committee may reach one of five conclusions:

1 to admonish the doctor;

2 to postpone a decision in order to collect more evidence;

3 to place conditions on the registration of the doctor for up to 3 years;

4 to suspend the registration of the doctor for up to a year; or

5 to erase the registration of the doctor.

There is a right of appeal if the doctor considers the conclusion to be incorrect.

Chapter four

The Medico-legal Aspects of Mental Disease

Normal and abnormal behaviour
Types of abnormal mental condition
Mental health legislation and the criminal justice system

Criminal responsibility: age and mental capacity
The effect of drink or drugs on responsibility

Testamentary capacity

The interaction between mental health and criminal behaviour and the resulting contacts with the police, the criminal justice system and the prisons are extremely complex and most of this work lies within the specialist field of forensic psychiatry, but a general understanding of the law relating to mental health and criminal behaviour is essential for any medical practitioner.

NORMAL AND ABNORMAL BEHAVIOUR

The spectrum of behaviour that can be considered to be 'normal' depends on so many factors – national, cultural, social, ethical, religious etc. – that any definition of 'normality' must be extremely wide for any given population. A further complication is that 'abnormal behaviour' and behaviour due to 'disorders of the mind' are not one and the same thing, although the latter may be associated with the former. Not everyone whose behaviour is 'abnormal' is suffering from a 'disorder of the mind' and it is certainly untrue that everyone with a 'disorder of the mind' will behave 'abnormally'.

TYPES OF ABNORMAL MENTAL CONDITION

Mental abnormality can be congenital (mental defect, impairment, handicap or subnormality) or acquired

(mental disease or illness). These categories are not sharply divided, as diseases such as schizophrenia may have a congenital origin even if the manifestations are delayed and not all antisocial psychological traits can be classified as a disease.

The term mental subnormality covers a wide range of severity; for instance, individuals with Down's syndrome may, at one end of the spectrum, be able to attend normal school and go on to live an independent adult life. Mental subnormality *per se* generally has few criminal medico-legal aspects apart from for those individuals who may drift into crime: theft, such as shop-lifting, is most likely but arson and some sexual offences may be related, although there is no direct correlation between the mental state and these more serious offences. The old idea of a homicidal 'village idiot' is part of the mythology that used to be directed against those with mental subnormality.

The psychopathic personality is difficult to categorize into congenital or acquired, and the effects of nature and nurture are closely intertwined. In many ways, a psychopathic personality is not a mental defect at all but simply one extreme end of the spectrum of variation in individual personality. This trait is associated with a failure of maturation of the personality and the retention of a child-like selfishness. Frustration of any whim is not tolerated and may be met with immediate violence, including murder. The response to these acts of violence is completely devoid of any regret or remorse. However, these individuals may have no abnormality of thought, mood or intelligence.

True mental illnesses acquired or appearing after childhood comprise several major groups. Those that arise from some structural brain damage may be called organic psychoses, whereas those that appear to have no neurological basis are called functional psychoses.

The organic psychoses comprise the various dementias which may present with a bewildering constellation of signs and symptoms, of which lability of mood, failure of memory, deterioration of intellect, irritability, irrational anger, confusion and loss of social inhibitions are most likely to lead to some medico-legal consequences. The dementing or demented individual may well be arrested for unacceptable behaviour or even for sudden, inexplicable and uncharacteristic acts of violence. The aetiology of these dementias is very wide: multi-infarct dementia, infective, degenerative and metabolic disorders, direct physical trauma, the acute effects of toxic substances (e.g. carbon monoxide) and the effects of chronic ingestion of toxic substances (especially alcohol). Cerebral tumours, either primary or secondary, may also lead to rapid personality changes.

A few epileptics may occasionally have an identifiable organic basis for their disease and some may have a concomitant mental abnormality. Of greater medico-legal interest are the rare episodes of post-ictal automatism and some forms of pre-fit aura, which may, rarely, give rise to dangerous behaviour.

The functional psychoses are characterized by disorders of thought for which no discernible physical basis can be identified and which can be seen as severe exaggerations of the normal variations of mood experienced by everyone. The functional psychoses are further subdivided into the affective psychoses, in which disorders of mood (affect) are the prime feature, and schizophrenic psychoses, in which disorders of the thought process are dominant.

A severe example of an affective disorder is the individual with manic–depressive psychosis who shows wide swings of mood from euphoric elation and hyperactivity to deepest depression and stupor. These changes in mood are quite out of proportion or often totally unrelated to external circumstances; however, for most of the time the individual will remain in some sort of equilibrium between the two extremes.

In the schizophrenic psychoses there are commonly delusions, mistaken beliefs held by the patient that cannot be altered by logical argument, and also hallucinations, which are false sensory experiences without true sensory stimuli. Patients may also have illusions, which are real sensory perceptions that are misinterpreted as something quite different. Commonly, these individuals have lost contact with reality.

The forensic aspects of these severe mental illnesses depend on the type and severity of the disease. On the one hand are the increased suicides that are associated with all forms of psychosis, and the confusion inherent in a manic–depressive psychosis may also apparently manifest itself in petty theft, especially shop-lifting.

Schizophrenics may sometimes be even more dangerous to their family or their immediate circle as they cannot see the real world clearly, if at all, because their thought processes are distorted by delusions, illusions and hallucinations. For instance, they may decide to 'rescue' someone from the harm or dangers that they falsely perceive by a 'mercy killing'. These fantasies may obstruct their normal living activities, often monopolizing their attention to the exclusion of real practicalities. In paranoid schizophrenia, the delusions and hallucinations are of a persecutory nature and the victims spend their lives in suspicious analysis of every event around them, and these feelings can be aggravated by hallucinations of voices and whispering and pseudo-scientific fears of malign rays and electronic surveillance.

In another clinical manifestation, the schizophrenic may become withdrawn, apathetic and sometimes neglectful and dirty, which may reach extremes at which the individual is catatonic. These individuals seldom cause harm to others, but may need protection from themselves and their illness.

Most commonly, schizophrenics have difficulty in surviving unaided in modern society; they may be unemployable, adopt a vagrant lifestyle and resort to petty theft and deceptions, but only very few will commit more serious crimes, including assaults and homicide. That most of the notorious multiple murderers are claimed to be schizophrenic or to have 'schizophrenic tendencies' possibly owes more to their defence strategy than to a strictly applied and universally accepted clinical diagnosis.

MENTAL HEALTH LEGISLATION AND THE CRIMINAL JUSTICE SYSTEM

Most advanced countries have legislation that allows for the detention and treatment of individuals, against their will, if they are diagnosed to have such severe mental disorders that they are a danger to themselves or to the public. The individual with mental health problems may also come into contact with doctors through various stages of the criminal justice system.

In the UK, if the police officer in charge of detainees in the custody suite is concerned about the physical or mental health of an individual, he may request that they are assessed by a doctor with expertise in clinical forensic medicine – known in the UK as a Forensic Medical Examiner (FME) or a police surgeon – at the police station. The FME will be asked to confirm that the detainee is 'fit to be detained' within the police station and also that he is 'fit to be interviewed'. During these examinations, the mental health of the individual will come under scrutiny. Rarely, it will be apparent that the detainee has a serious mental illness that requires urgent treatment in a secure hospital environment; more commonly, some less serious disease is identified that may require treatment either in hospital or while the individual is detained at the police station.

An individual may be considered to be unfit for interview for a number of reasons, amongst which is mental deficiency or illness. If an individual is not considered to be 'fit to be interviewed', for whatever reason, the police cannot interview him and this provides a very important point of protection for what might be a vulnerable individual. In some cases of mental deficiency or illness, an 'appropriate adult' (social worker etc.) may be appointed to be present during the interviews to ensure that no undue pressure or influence is brought to bear on an individual with mental health problems.

CRIMINAL RESPONSIBILITY: AGE AND MENTAL CAPACITY

All advanced countries accept that children under a certain age should not be held criminally responsible for their actions. This age of responsibility varies in different countries but in England, for example, no child under 10 years can be held responsible for any act, even if it is obviously criminal. The law holds that the child below 10 years is too immature to have the *mens rea* or 'guilty mind' (meaning intent) that lays a person open to account for his antisocial acts, and no attempt may be made to show that the child knew the evil nature of his behaviour. Children aged between

10 and 13 are now considered to be capable of distinguishing between serious wrong and simple naughtiness and children of this age are now treated in the same way as juveniles aged 14 to 17 years.

Similarly, most legal systems have provision for excusing an adult who, by reason of mental defect or abnormality, commits what would otherwise be a criminal act. The problem lies in determining what is a sufficient degree of mental abnormality to qualify for this exclusion from the retribution of the law. Every country has its own criteria for evaluating the degree of mental impairment that will excuse criminal responsibility: the English legal system has been used as the basis for the legal systems in many parts of the world, although it must be noted that the concept of 'diminished responsibility', introduced into English law as late as 1957, was copied from Scotland, where it had already been in use for a very long period.

Unfitness to plead indicates a severe degree of mental disease, the type being immaterial, which would cause the accused person to be unfit to appear at a criminal trial. It does not matter if the person had been perfectly normal at the time of committing the offence – it is his condition at the time of trial that is relevant. It would be against natural justice to stand a person in court if he was incapable of appreciating what was happening to him. For a person to be 'unfit to plead' it must be shown that he would be unable by reason of his mental illness:

- to understand the nature of the court proceedings;
- to understand what he was being accused of and why he was there;
- to challenge any of the jurors, as is his normal right;
- to instruct the lawyers acting in his defence.

The degree of abnormality has to be quite profound for people to be unfit to plead; they are often deluded, confused or in profound depression bordering on stupor. If this plea is accepted, the defendant can then only be committed to a secure mental hospital for an indefinite period, though should he recover he could theoretically be brought back for trial.

When the defendant is fit to plead, the only way in which criminal responsibility can be evaded is by proving the existence of a 'sufficient' mental abnormality. Until the concept of diminished responsibility was introduced, the term 'sufficient' meant that the mental disorder had to be severe enough for the verdict at the trial to be that the accused was 'guilty but insane' at the time of the offence. Such a verdict automatically led to committal to a criminal mental institution for an indefinite period and so it was only of assistance to the defendant in cases of murder.

In 1957 the Homicide Act introduced the concept of 'diminished responsibility' which, in part, was intended as a means of avoiding the death sentence for people with a lesser degree of mental abnormality than could be brought within the McNaghten Rules, which were the former test of 'sufficient' mental disease. However, as capital punishment was abolished in Britain soon after the introduction of the Act, this change lost much of its force, as a sentence of life imprisonment (nominally 15 years but in reality only about 10 years in prison) would be less than an indefinite stay in a criminal mental hospital.

The Homicide Act states that:

Where a person kills another, he shall not be convicted of murder if he was suffering from such abnormality of mind (whether arising from a condition of arrested development or any inherent causes or induced by disease or injury) as substantially impaired his mental responsibility for his acts and omissions in doing or being a party to the killing.

The wording of the Act makes no effort to quantify or describe the 'abnormality of mind', this being left to the expert medical witnesses involved in the case. The Homicide Act also allows extenuation for provocation, 'whether by things done or things said or by both together', that may cause a person to lose his self-control. This assessment is not a matter for experts and is left to the jury.

In practice, the defendant will usually be examined by a specialist forensic psychiatrist on behalf of the state and may also be examined by specialist psychiatrists retained by the defence. In some murder trials, when the actual facts of the killing are not in dispute, the only evidence offered may be the psychiatric medical evidence.

THE EFFECT OF DRINK OR DRUGS ON RESPONSIBILITY

In general, the effect of alcohol or of any drugs on a person is no excuse for his criminal actions. If a person voluntarily gets drunk or 'high' on drugs, any subsequent criminal act is his responsibility as he is supposed to be aware that drink or drugs have the potential to affect his

behaviour. However, if he can prove that these were not taken voluntarily, for example that someone else has slipped strong drink into a coffee or a beer, there is a possible defence.

In more serious crimes, usually homicide, it has been pleaded that the state of intoxication was so severe that the accused was rendered incapable of forming any intent to kill and therefore could not have the *mens rea* or 'guilty mind' which is the essence of culpability in a normal adult. This defence is accepted with great reluctance, as is amnesia, the claim that no recollection of the events remains.

TESTAMENTARY CAPACITY

Mental illness may affect matters of civil as well as criminal law. In Britain the law defines the capacity to make a will as the 'possession of a sound disposing mind'. It is not concerned with whether the testator (the person making the will) is suffering from some mental illness, but merely with whether, at the time they are about to make their will:

- they know of what property they possess and how they are able to dispose of it – that is, they know what a will is;
- they know to whom they may reasonably give their possessions and the nature of the formality they are about to carry out;
- they have some good reason for their actions – not being obsessed with some unreasonable dislike or affected by delusions which prevent a sense of right or wrong.

If a person is unable to speak, he may signify his approval or otherwise of questions put to him by a nod or shake of his head and so is not prevented by this disability from making a will. He must appear to understand the purport of the questions dealing with the disposition of his property and, if this is so, he will be considered legally to possess a sound testamentary capacity. Under English law, if people cannot fulfil these criteria, a judge can authorize another person to make a will on their behalf.

That there must be no undue influence by any other person on a testator is self-evident, but unfortunately in the past there have been some substantiated allegations that medical attendants around a sick or dying person have influenced him in their favour in the disposition of his property after death. To establish undue influence, it is necessary to prove coercion or some kind of fraud.

The will must be signed at the end by two witnesses who are present at the same time and who saw the testator actually sign his name. They do not have to be aware of the contents of the will, only the fact of signing. Even a mark by the testator, if he is too ill to write, is sufficient and he may direct that some other person signs for him; clearly, the witnesses must confirm that this request has been made when they witness the signing of the will.

A doctor is often called upon to be one of the two witnesses of the signing of a will and he may later be a valuable witness if the will is subsequently contested by dissatisfied relatives who may wish to establish that it was made while the testator was of unsound mind or that undue influence was exerted on him. Death may take place years after the will was made and the doctor who witnessed the signature can be called upon to give evidence as to the capacity of the testator if the matter proceeds to court for trial. Neither an attesting witness nor his or her spouse can receive a gift from the will.

Chapter five

The Medical Aspects of Death

Death is such a common feature of medical practice that all doctors will have come into contact with it at some time in their medical career.

DEFINITION OF DEATH

It is only organisms that have experienced life that can die, because death is the cessation of life in a previously living organism. A rock cannot die because it has never lived, but the fossil contained within it has lived and has died. Medically and scientifically, death is not an event, it is a process, and this is particularly so in the higher animals, including humans, in which the more complex and more specialized internal organs have different functions with different cellular metabolic processes which cease to function at different rates.

This differential rate of cellular death has resulted in much debate – ethical, religious and moral – as to when 'death' actually occurs. The practical solution to this argument is to consider the death of a single cell (cellular death) and the cessation of the integrated functioning of an individual (somatic death) as two separate aspects.

Cellular death

Cellular death means the cessation of respiration (the utilization of oxygen) and the normal metabolic activity in the body tissues and cells. Cessation of respiration is soon followed by autolysis and decay, which, if it affects the whole body, is indisputable evidence of true death. The differences in cellular metabolism determine the rate with which cells die and this can be very variable – except, perhaps, in the synchronous death of all of the cells following a nearby nuclear explosion.

Skin and bone will remain metabolically active and thus 'alive' for many hours and these cells can be successfully cultured days after somatic death. White blood cells are capable of movement for up to 12 hours after cardiac arrest – a fact that makes the concept of microscopic identification of a 'vital reaction' to injury of doubtful reliability. The cortical neuron, on the other hand, will die after only 3–7 minutes of complete oxygen deprivation. A body dies cell by cell and the complete process may take many hours.

Somatic death

Somatic death means that the individual will never again communicate or deliberately interact with the environment. The individual is irreversibly unconscious and unaware of both the world and his own existence. The key word in this definition is 'irreversible', as lack of communication and interaction with the environment may also occur during deep sleep, under anaesthesia and as a result of a temporary coma. Even if irreversible unconsciousness has occurred, if there continues to be spontaneous respiratory movements and the heart continues to beat, it is doubtful if this would be accepted as fulfilling the criteria of 'true death'.

RESUSCITATION

Advances in resuscitation techniques, in ventilation and in the support of the unconscious patient have resulted in the survival of patients who would otherwise have died as a result of direct cerebral trauma or of cerebral hypoxia from whatever cause. There is a spectrum of survival: some will recover both spontaneous respiration and consciousness, others will never regain consciousness but will regain the ability to breathe on their own, and some will regain neither consciousness nor the ability to breathe and will require permanent artificial ventilation to remain 'alive'.

The Department of Health in the UK, acting on advice from a Conference of the Royal Colleges, published a definitive Code of Practice in the 1970s concerning the diagnosis of brain death and this code is now accepted both legally and medically as being reliable. The main points are:

- The patient must be in deep coma and treatable causes such as depressant drugs, metabolic or endocrine disorders (diabetic or myxoedema coma) or hypothermia must be excluded.
- The patient must be on mechanical ventilation because of absent or inadequate spontaneous respiration. Neuromuscular blocking agents and any curare-like drugs must be excluded as a possible cause of the respiratory failure.
- A firm diagnosis of the basic pathology must be available and must be known to be due to irremediable brain damage. The most common causes are head injury and intracerebral haemorrhage from a ruptured cerebral aneurysm.

- Diagnostic tests for brainstem death must be unequivocally positive. These tests should be determined by two doctors, preferably one of whom should be the physician in charge of the patient. This physician should have been registered for at least 5 years and should have had experience of such cases. The second, independent doctor should have similar experience. If there has been a request for organ donation, none of the doctors involved in the care of the patient or in the final diagnosis of brainstem death may be part of the transplant team.
- A checklist of the diagnostic tests and their results should be kept in the patient's notes and the tests should be repeated at least once, the interval between the tests depending on the opinion of the doctors.

In order to establish the points of the Code of Practice in the UK, a series of clinical tests must be performed and these are set out below. In other jurisdictions, additional tests, including electroencephalography and even cerebral angiography or cerebral blood flow measurements, are required.

- All brainstem reflexes are absent, with fixed dilated and unreactive pupils. Corneal reflexes are absent. It should be noted that persistence of spinal reflexes are irrelevant in the diagnosis of brainstem death.
- Vestibulo-ocular reflexes are negative when iced water is introduced into the ears.
- There are no motor responses to painful stimuli in any of the cranial nerves.
- There is no gag reflex to a catheter placed in the larynx and trachea.
- There are no respiratory movements when the patient is disconnected from the ventilator with an arterial P_{CO_2} level in excess of 50 mmHg as a stimulus to breathing.
- Testing must be performed with a body temperature not less then 35°C to avoid hypothermia simulating brainstem damage.

Advances in resuscitation and ventilation techniques now prevent the immediate death of many individuals. Previously, brainstem death would lead inexorably to respiratory arrest and this would cause myocardial hypoxia and cardiac arrest. Artificial ventilation breaks that chain and, while ventilation is continued, myocardial hypoxia and cardiac arrest are prevented.

PERSISTENT VEGETATIVE STATE

Developments in the care of the long-term uncon-scious patient, particularly their nutrition, led to the long-term survival of the unconscious but spontan-eously respiring patient. The term persistent vegeta-tive state (PVS) was coined to describe this condition, in which it is assumed there is some functioning brainstem activity but no higher cerebral function can be detected. It has long been accepted that medical treatment in terms of drug therapy, antibiotics etc. can be withdrawn if there is no chance of survival, this usually being done after discussion with the relatives. The position with regard to PVS patients is slightly different: they are not in need of life-sustaining treat-ment and, unless they develop a chest infection, they do not require antibiotics. What they do require is nutrition and hydration.

This situation was considered by the English courts in 1993 when they reviewed the case of Tony Bland, a young man who suffered crush (traumatic) asphyxia causing cerebral hypoxia at the Hillsborough football crowd disaster some 2 years earlier. His parents asked for nutrition be withdrawn, allowing their son to die with dignity. The court gave consent to the withdrawal of nutrition and Tony Bland died a week or so later. Other cases have followed and the courts have con-sidered each on its own merits. If, however, the rela-tives wish to withdraw treatment and nutrition in the knowledge that this will lead to death, the court is most unlikely to refuse their request, providing a diag-nosis of PVS is confirmed.

TISSUE AND ORGAN TRANSPLANTATION

The laws relating to tissue and organ donation and transplantation are dependent upon the religious and ethical views of the country in which they apply. The laws vary in both extent and detail around the world, but there are very few countries where transplantation is expressly forbidden and few religions that forbid it – Jehovah's Witnesses are one such group, who also reject transfusion of donated blood.

The organs and tissues to be transplanted may come from one of several sources.

Homologous transplantation

Tissue is moved between sites on the same body. For instance, skin is taken from the thigh to graft onto a burn site or bone chips from the pelvis may be taken to assist in the healing of the fragmented fracture site of a long bone. Homologous blood transfusion can be used where there is a religious objection to the use of anonymously donated blood.

Live donation

In this process, tissue is taken from a living donor whose tissues have been matched to or are compatible with those of the recipient. The most common example is blood transfusion but marrow transplantation is now also very common. Other live donations usually involve the kidneys as these are paired organs and donors can, if the remaining kidney is healthy, maintain their elec-trolyte and water balance with only one kidney.

Most kidneys for transplant are derived from cadaveric donation (see below), but live donation is also possible and this, associated with a high demand for kidneys, especially in Western countries, has resulted in a few surgeons seeking donors (in particular poor people from developing countries) who would be will-ing to sell one of their kidneys. This practice is illegal in many countries and, if not specifically illegal, it is certainly unethical.

With increasing surgical skill, the transplantation of a part of a singleton organ with large physiological reserve (such as the liver) has been attempted. These transplants are not as successful as the whole organ transplants and the risks to the donor are considerably higher.

Cadaveric donation

In many countries, cadaveric donation is the major source of all tissues for transplantation. The surgical techniques to harvest the organs are improving, as are the storage and transportation techniques, but the best results are still obtained if the organs are obtained while circulation is present or immediately after cessa-tion of the circulation. The aim being to minimize the 'warm ischaemic time', kidneys are more resilient to anoxia than some other organs and can survive up to 30 minutes after cardiac stoppage.

Cadaveric donation is now so well established that most developed countries have sophisticated laws to regulate it. However, these laws vary greatly: some countries allow the removal of organs no matter what the wishes of the relatives, other countries allow for an 'opting-out' process in which organs can be taken for transplantation unless there is an objection from relatives. The converse of that system is the one practised in the UK, which requires 'opting in'. In this system, the transplant team must ensure that the donor either gave active permission during life or at least did not object and also that no close relative objects after death. The Human Tissue Act (1961, and in Northern Ireland 1962) allows the person 'in lawful possession' of a body to authorize the donation of tissues or organs only if he has no reason to believe that (a) the deceased had indicated during life that he objected to donation and that (b) the surviving spouse or relative of the deceased objects.

If an autopsy will be required by law for any reason, the permission of the Coroner, Procurator Fiscal or other legal officer investigating the death must be obtained before harvesting of tissue or organs is undertaken. In general, there is seldom any reason for the legal officer investigating the death to object to organ or tissue donation because it is self-evident that injured, diseased or damaged organs are unlikely to be harvested and certainly will not be transplanted and so will be available for examination. In what is almost always a tragic unexpected death, the donation of organs may be the one positive feature and can often be of great assistance to the relatives.

Xenografts

Grafting of animal tissue into humans has always seemed tempting and clinical trials have been performed with limited success. There is considerable difficulty with cross-matching the tissues and considerable concern about the possibility of transfer of animal viruses to an immunocompromised human host. Strains of donor animals, usually pigs, are being bred in clinically clean conditions to prevent viral contamination, but there is still no guarantee of a close or ideal tissue match. Also, the complexity of their breeding and rearing means that these animals are expensive.

Cloning

A potentially cheaper solution involves the cloning of animals for use as transplant donors. This research took a step forward with the successful cloning of Dolly the sheep, but other advances have been slow to appear and although cloning remains a theoretical course of action, much research is still to be done.

DEATH CERTIFICATION

Exactly how a doctor determines death is a matter of individual, local, national and international choice. Some simply palpate for pulse and respiration, some require absence of heart sounds and breath sounds on auscultation, some require a flat trace on an ECG.

In general, if a doctor knows the cause of death and the cause of death is natural and without any suspicious or unusual features, he may issue a certificate of the medical cause of death – commonly called a death certificate. Which doctor may do this varies: in some countries the doctor must have seen and treated the patient before death, whereas in other countries any doctor who has seen the body after death may issue a certificate.

The format of certifying the cause of death is now defined by the World Health Organization (WHO) and is an international standard that is now used in most countries. The system divides the cause of death into two parts: the first part (Part I) describes the condition(s) that led directly to death; Part II is for other conditions, not related to those listed in Part I, that have also contributed to death.

Part I is divided into subsections and generally three – (a), (b) and (c) – are printed on the certificate. These subsections are for disease processes that have led directly to death and that are causally related to one another, (a) being due to or consequent on (b), which in turn is due to or consequent on (c). It is important to realize that, in this system of death certification, it is the disease lowest in the Part I list that is the most important, as it is the primary pathological condition, the start of the events leading to death. It is this disease that is most important statistically and is used to compile national and international mortality statistics.

It is not necessary to complete parts Ib, Ic or II if there are no predisposing conditions; it is sufficient to

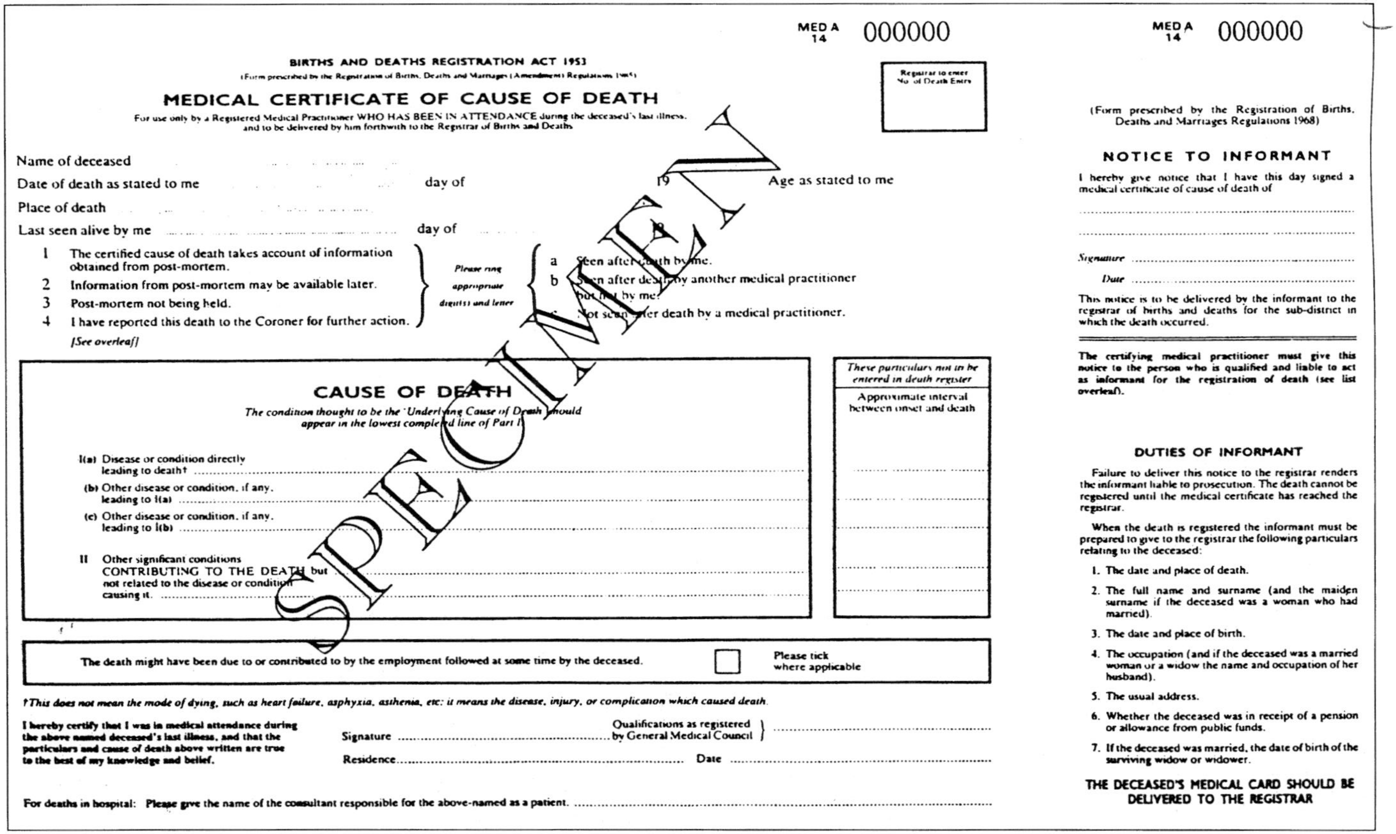
MED A 14 000000

BIRTHS AND DEATHS REGISTRATION ACT 1953

(Form prescribed by the Registration of Births, Deaths and Marriages (Amendment) Regulations 1985)

MEDICAL CERTIFICATE OF CAUSE OF DEATH

For use only by a Registered Medical Practitioner WHO HAS BEEN IN ATTENDANCE during the deceased's last illness, and to be delivered by him forthwith to the Registrar of Births and Deaths

Registrar to enter No. of Death Entry

Name of deceased

Date of death as stated to me .... day of .... 19 .... Age as stated to me

Place of death

Last seen alive by me .... day of 19

1 The certified cause of death takes account of information obtained from post-mortem.
2 Information from post-mortem may be available later.
3 Post-mortem not being held.
4 I have reported this death to the Coroner for further action.
[See overleaf]

Please ring appropriate digit(s) and letter

a Seen after death by me.
b Seen after death by another medical practitioner but not by me.
c Not seen after death by a medical practitioner.

CAUSE OF DEATH

The condition thought to be the 'Underlying Cause of Death' should appear in the lowest completed line of Part I.

I(a) Disease or condition directly leading to death† ....
(b) Other disease or condition, if any, leading to I(a) ....
(c) Other disease or condition, if any, leading to I(b) ....

II Other significant conditions CONTRIBUTING TO THE DEATH but not related to the disease or condition causing it. ....

These particulars not to be entered in death register

Approximate interval between onset and death

The death might have been due to or contributed to by the employment followed at some time by the deceased. ☐ Please tick where applicable

†This does not mean the mode of dying, such as heart failure, asphyxia, asthenia, etc: it means the disease, injury, or complication which caused death.

I hereby certify that I was in medical attendance during the above named deceased's last illness, and that the particulars and cause of death above written are true to the best of my knowledge and belief.

Signature .... Qualifications as registered by General Medical Council ....

Residence .... Date ....

For deaths in hospital: Please give the name of the consultant responsible for the above-named as a patient. ....

MED A 14 000000

(Form prescribed by the Registration of Births, Deaths and Marriages Regulations 1968)

NOTICE TO INFORMANT

I hereby give notice that I have this day signed a medical certificate of cause of death of

....

Signature ....

Date ....

This notice is to be delivered by the informant to the registrar of births and deaths for the sub-district in which the death occurred.

The certifying medical practitioner must give this notice to the person who is qualified and liable to act as informant for the registration of death (see list overleaf).

DUTIES OF INFORMANT

Failure to deliver this notice to the registrar renders the informant liable to prosecution. The death cannot be registered until the medical certificate has reached the registrar.

When the death is registered the informant must be prepared to give to the registrar the following particulars relating to the deceased:

1. The date and place of death.
2. The full name and surname (and the maiden surname if the deceased was a woman who had married).
3. The date and place of birth.
4. The occupation (and if the deceased was a married woman or a widow the name and occupation of her husband).
5. The usual address.
6. Whether the deceased was in receipt of a pension or allowance from public funds.
7. If the deceased was married, the date of birth of the surviving widow or widower.

THE DECEASED'S MEDICAL CARD SHOULD BE DELIVERED TO THE REGISTRAR

SPECIMEN

Figure 5.1 Reproduction of death certificate (doctor's counterfoil omitted).

record the cause of death, for example as:

Ia Intracerebral haemorrhage

Alternatively, if the same patient survived for a number of days or weeks before succumbing to a chest infection, the death certificate should record both processes:

Ia Bronchopneumonia
Ib Intracerebral haemorrhage

Statistically, both certificates would record the primary disease as intracerebral haemorrhage.

Doctors should resist including the mode of death (coma, heart failure etc.) on the death certificate; these terms are not prohibited but they are not useful. Thus:

Ia Heart failure
Ib Hypertrophic cardiomyopathy

or:

Ia Coma
Ib Subarachnoid haemorrhage
Ic Ruptured congenital aneurysm

are not incorrect, they are just overly cumbersome.

All too often, doctors give only a mode of death without documenting the underlying pathology or specific disease process; this may represent the main clinical symptoms but has no statistical significance whatever.

Some jurisdictions will allow specific causes of death that would not be acceptable elsewhere. In the UK it is acceptable, if the patient is over 70 years of age, to record 'Ia: Old age'.

Some doctors would limit this conclusion to those patients who died after a slow and inexorable decline but, in the absence of any specific diagnosis, others may be tempted to use it for any individual over the minimum age limit, even in the face of an established diagnosis of a lethal disease.

At the other end of the age range, the diagnosis of sudden infant death syndrome is now well established; unfortunately, the diagnostic criteria are seldom as well known and even less frequently are they applied to the letter.

The second part of the death certificate is often more problematical and is commonly used as something of a 'dustbin' to record all, many or some of the diseases afflicting the patient at the time of death. Part II is most often used for the elderly in whom multiple pathologies may well have contributed to death.

Death certificates are important documents but the information on them may be unreliable for the reasons discussed above or they may be incomplete or incorrect because the doctor chooses not to complete them in full deliberately to give false information. The former may occur when the doctor does not want members of the family to discover the disease(s) from which the patient died. This is most common in sexually transmitted diseases – once it was syphilis now it is AIDS. The latter occurs when a doctor is dishonest; he may be hiding his clinical incompetence or, worse, he may be concealing a homicide.

International classifications of disease are now well established and the WHO produces a book, *International Classification of Disease* (ICD), which can be used for both clinical diagnoses and death certificates. In this classification, each condition is given a four-digit ICD code, which simplifies both data recording and data analysis and allows information from many national and international sources to be compared.

In some countries, doctors also have to record the manner of death (homicide, suicide etc.) on the death certificate, as advocated by the WHO; however, in most Western countries with an efficient medico-legal investigative system, the conclusion about the manner of death is delegated to a legal officer – this may be the Coroner in England and Wales, the Procurator Fiscal in Scotland, the Medical Examiner in some of the states of the USA, a magistrate etc.

MEDICO-LEGAL INVESTIGATION OF DEATH

If a death is natural and a doctor can sign a death certificate, this allows the relatives to continue with the process of disposal of the body, whether by burial or cremation. If the death is not natural or if no doctor can complete a death certificate, some other method of investigating and certifying the death must be present. In England and Wales there are approximately 560 000 deaths each year, of which about 435 000 are certified by doctors, but some 55 000 of these cases are only certified after discussion with the coroner's office. The coroners themselves certify some 122 000 deaths a year and most usually require an autopsy examination before doing so.

The deaths that cannot be certified by a doctor are examined by a variety of legal officers in other countries: coroners, procurators fiscal, medical examiners, magistrates, judges and even police officers. The exact systems of referral, responsibility and investigation

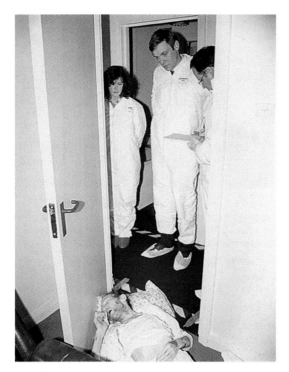

Figure 5.2 The pathologist, forensic medical examiner and senior police officer at the scene of a sudden death. Face masks would now be worn to prevent DNA contamination of the scene.

differ widely, but the general framework is much the same. The systems are arranged to identify and investigate deaths that are, or might be, unnatural and that might be overtly criminal, suspicious, traumatic or due to poisoning or that might simply be deaths that are unexpected or unexplained.

There is no common law duty for a doctor to report an unnatural death to the coroner, but it would perhaps be a foolish or foolhardy doctor who did not do so. Conversely, the Registrar of Deaths does have a duty to inform the coroner about any death that appears to be unnatural or where the rules about completion of the death certificate have not been complied with.

Following the death of a person who has not been receiving medical supervision and where no doctor was in attendance, the fact of death can be confirmed by nurses, paramedics and other healthcare professionals as well as by doctors. The police will usually investigate the scene and the circumstances of the death and report their findings to the coroner or other legal authority. The coroner, through his officers, will attempt to find a family practitioner to obtain medical details. That family practitioner, if found, may be able to complete the death certificate if he is aware of sufficient natural disease and if the scene and circumstances of the death are not suspicious.

If no family practitioner can be found, or if the practitioner is unwilling to issue a death certificate, the coroner will usually exercise his right to request an autopsy, but in Scotland the ability to perform only an external examination of the body on cases such as this – the so-called 'view and grant'– is well established.

This all-embracing coronial power to order autopsies is not found in other countries, where autopsies are often much more restricted. It is not surprising, therefore, that the autopsy rate varies widely from jurisdiction to jurisdiction; in some cases it is nearly 100 per cent but it may fall as low as 5–10 per cent. Some jurisdictions with low autopsy rates insist on the external examination of the body by a doctor with medico-legal training. Autopsy examinations are not the complete and final answer to every death, but without an internal examination it can be impossible to be certain about the cause and the mechanism of death. It should be remembered that at least 50 per cent of the causes of death given by doctors have been shown to be incorrect by a subsequent autopsy.

In England and Wales, the coroner may take an interest in any body lying within his jurisdiction, whether referred or not. However, most cases are referred to the coroner by doctors, police and members of the public. Deaths may also be referred by the Registrar of Deaths if a death certificate issued by a doctor is unacceptable, which it may be for the following reasons:

- the deceased was not attended in his last illness by the doctor completing the certificate;
- the deceased had not been seen by a doctor either after death or within 14 days prior to death;
- where the cause of death is unknown;
- where death appears to be due to poisoning or to industrial disease;
- where death may have been unnatural or where it may have been caused by violence or neglect or abortion or where it is associated with suspicious circumstances;
- where death occurred during a surgical operation or before recovery from an anaesthetic.

Once a death is reported the coroner, if he is satisfied that it is due to natural causes, he can decide not to pursue any further enquiries and to ask the doctor to issue a death certificate. Alternatively, and more commonly, he may order an autopsy and, if this reveals that death was due to natural causes, may issue a certificate to allow for disposal of the body. If the autopsy cannot establish that death was due to natural causes or if there is a public interest in the death, the coroner may hold an inquest – a public inquiry into the death. The modern inquest is severely restricted in its functions and the verdicts it may return. An inquest seeks to answer four questions: who the person is, when and where they died and how they died. The 'who', 'when' and 'where' questions seldom pose a problem; it is the answer to the fourth question – the 'how' – that is often the most difficult.

The coroner can sit with or without a jury, except in some specific cases (e.g. deaths on a rail-track or in a prison) when they must sit with a jury. The coroner's court cannot form any view about either criminal or civil blame for the death. Indeed, some would say that the coroners' system is long overdue for the review that is currently taking place.

A coroner or the jury has a prescribed list of possible verdicts and, although riders or comments may be attached to these verdicts, they must not indicate or imply blame. The commonly used verdicts include:

- Unlawful killing (which includes murder, manslaughter, infanticide, death by dangerous driving etc.);
- Lawful killing (legal use of lethal force by a police officer);
- Accident (misadventure);
- Killed himself/herself (suicide);
- Natural causes;
- Industrial disease;
- Abuse of drugs (dependent or non-dependent);
- Open verdict (where the evidence is insufficient to reach any other verdict).

THE AUTOPSY

The words autopsy, necropsy and post-mortem examination are synonymous, although post-mortem examination can have a broader meaning encompassing any examination made after death, including a simple external examination. In general terms, autopsies can be performed for two reasons: clinical interest and medico-legal purposes.

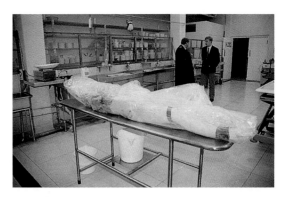

Figure 5.3 A body found in suspicious circumstances must be protected during the journey from scene to mortuary to preserve any trace evidence. Body bags are commonly used, but here the body has been wrapped in plastic sheeting.

The clinical autopsy is performed in a hospital mortuary after consent for the examination has been sought from and granted by the relatives of the deceased. The doctors treating the patient should know why their patient has died and be able to complete a death certificate even in the absence of an autopsy. These examinations have been used in the past for the teaching of medical students etc. and for research.

The medico-legal autopsy is performed on behalf of the state. The aims of these examinations are much broader than those of the clinical autopsy and include:

- to identity of the body;
- to estimate the time of death;
- to identify and document the nature and number of injuries;
- to interpret the significance and effect of the injuries;
- to identify the presence of any natural disease;
- to interpret the significance and effect of the natural disease present;
- to identify the presence of poisons; and
- to interpret the effect of any medical or surgical treatment.

Taken at its broadest, autopsies can be performed by any doctor, but ideally they should be performed by a properly trained pathologist. Medico-legal autopsies are a specialized version of the standard autopsy and should be performed by pathologists who have had the necessary training and experience in forensic pathology. The autopsy should be performed in a mortuary with adequate facilities. (Guidelines for an autopsy are contained in Appendix 1.)

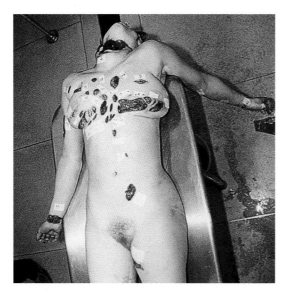

Figure 5.4 Where multiple wounds are present, numbering the individual injuries will assist in relating them to the autopsy report. Note the variation in the appearances of these stab wounds, all inflicted by the same knife.

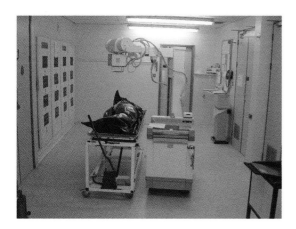

Figure 5.5 Radiology is essential in some autopsies.

However, where there are no trained staff or no adequate facilities – which can occur not only in some developing countries but also in some so-called developed countries that do not adequately fund their medico-legal systems – non-specialist doctors may occasionally have to perform autopsies and histopathologists may have to perform medico-legal autopsies. A poorly performed autopsy may be considerably worse than no autopsy at all; it is certainly worse than

an autopsy delayed for a short while to await the arrival of a specialist.

The first crucial part of any autopsy is observation and documentation and these skills should lie within the competence of almost every doctor. All documentation should be in writing, and diagrams, drawings and annotations must be signed and dated at the end of the examination. Photographs are extremely useful and, if used, should always include a scale and some anatomical reference point.

EXHUMATION

It is rare for a body to be removed from its grave for further examination; the most common reasons for exhumation are personal, for example if a family chooses to move the body or if a cemetery is to be closed or altered. Various legal formalities must be observed before permission to exhume a body can be given, but these lie outside the scope of this book. Once legal permission has been given, the correct site of the grave must be determined from plans and records of the cemetery as well as inscriptions on headstones.

In some countries with a low autopsy rate, for example Belgium, exhumations are more common, as legal arguments about an accident or an insurance claim etc. require an examination of the body to establish the medical facts.

The mechanics of removal of a coffin require some thought and the practice of actually lifting the coffin before dawn owes more to Hollywood than to practical needs. Because the body may need to be examined as quickly as possible due to decomposition, the mortuary, the pathologist, the police and everyone else with a legitimate interest must be aware of the time arranged.

An examination of a body after exhumation is seldom as good as the examination of a fresh body, but it is surprising how well preserved a body may remain and how useful such an examination often is. It is almost impossible to predict how well preserved a body might be, as there are so many confounding factors. The autopsy that follows an exhumation is basically the same as that performed at any other time, although decomposition may lead to some modification of the basic technique. Exhumations are the province of the skilled and experienced forensic pathologist.

If there is a possibility that poisoning may have played a part in the death, samples of soil should be taken from above, below and to the sides of the coffin and submitted for toxicological examination. A control sample should also be taken from a distant part of the cemetery. Additional samples should be taken of any fluid or solid material within the coffin. In fact, this is only of significance in arsenic poisoning, but these control samples may prove useful if any suggestion of contamination is raised at a later date.

Chapter six

Changes after Death

It is accepted by everyone that if irreversible cardiac arrest has occurred, the individual has died and eventually all of the cells of the body will cease their normal metabolic functions and the changes of decomposition will begin. Initially these changes can only be detected biochemically as the metabolism in the cells alters to autolytic pathways. Eventually the changes become visible and these visible changes are important for two reasons: firstly, because a doctor needs to know the normal progress of decomposition so that he does not misinterpret these normal changes for signs of an unnatural death and, secondly, because they can be used in determining how long the individual has been dead.

EARLY CHANGES

When the heart stops and breathing ceases, there is an immediate fall in blood pressure and the supply of oxygen to the cells of the body ceases. Initially the cells that can use anoxic pathways will do so until their metabolic reserves are exhausted, and then their metabolism will begin to fail. With loss of neuronal activity, all nervous activity ceases, the reflexes are lost and breathing stops. In the eye the corneal reflex ceases and the pupils stop reacting to light. The retinal vessels, viewed with an ophthalmoscope, show the break up or fragmentation of the columns of blood, which is called 'trucking' or 'shunting' as the appearances have suggested the movement of railway wagons. The eyes themselves lose their intraocular tension.

The muscles rapidly become flaccid (primary flaccidity), with complete loss of tone, but they may retain their reactivity and may respond to touch and other forms of stimulation for some hours after cardiac arrest. Discharges of the dying motor neurons may stimulate small groups of muscle cells and lead to focal twitching, although these decrease with time.

The fall in blood pressure and cessation of circulation of the blood usually render the skin, conjunctivae and mucous membranes pale. The skin of the face and the lips may remain red or blue in colour in hypoxic/congestive deaths. The hair follicles die at the same time as the rest of the skin and there is no truth in the belief that hair continues to grow after death, although the beard may appear more prominent against a pale skin.

Loss of muscle tone in the sphincters may result in voiding of urine; this is such a common finding that no relationship with deaths from epilepsy or asphyxia can be established. Emission of semen is also found in some deaths; the presence of semen cannot be used as an indicator of sexual activity shortly before death.

Regurgitation is a very common feature of terminal collapse and it is a common complication of resuscitation. Gastric contents are identified in the mouth or airways in up to 25 per cent of all autopsies. The presence of this material cannot be used to indicate that inhalation was the cause of death unless it is supported by eyewitness accounts or by the microscopic identification of food debris in the peripheral airways.

RIGOR MORTIS

Rigor mortis is, at its simplest, a temperature-dependent physicochemical change that occurs within muscle cells as a result of lack of oxygen. The lack of oxygen means that energy cannot be obtained from glycogen via glucose using oxidative phosphorylation and so adenosine triphosphate (ATP) production from this process ceases and the secondary anoxic process takes over for a short time but, as lactic acid is a by-product of anoxic respiration, the cell cytoplasm becomes increasingly acidic. In the face of low ATP and high acidity, the actin and myosin fibres bind together and form a gel. The outward result of these complex cellular metabolic changes is that the muscles become stiff. However, they do not shorten unless they are under tension.

It is clear from the short discussion above that if muscle glycogen levels are low or if the muscle cells are acidic at the time of death as a result of exercise, the process of rigor will develop faster. Electrocution is also associated with rapidly developing rigor and this may be due to the repeated stimulation of the muscles. Conversely, in the young, the old or the emaciated, rigor may be extremely hard to detect because of the low muscle bulk.

Rigor develops uniformly throughout the body but it is first detectable in the smaller muscle groups such as those around the eyes and mouth, the jaw and the fingers. It appears to 'spread' down the body from the head to the legs as larger and larger muscle groups are rendered stiff.

The only use of assessing the presence or absence of rigor lies in the estimation of the time of death, and the key word here is 'estimation', as rigor is such a variable process that it can never provide an accurate assessment of the time of death and in practice should never be used alone. The chemical processes that result in the stiffening of the muscles, in common with all chemical processes, are affected by temperature: the colder the temperature the slower the reactions and vice versa. In a cold body, the onset of rigor will be delayed and the length of time that its effects on the muscles can be detected will be prolonged, whereas in a body lying in a warm environment, the onset of rigor and its duration will be short. It is important that forensic pathologists are aware of the normal time course of rigor for the country in which they practise.

It is also important to be aware of the microenvironment around the body when assessing rigor: a body lying in front of a fire or in a bath of hot water will develop rigor quickly, whereas rigor will progress slowly in a body lying outside in winter. When the post-mortem cooling of a body is extreme, the stiffening of the body may be due to the physical effects of cooling rather than rigor. This will become apparent when the body is moved to a warmer environment (usually the mortuary) and the stiffening due to cold is seen to disappear as the body warms. Continued observation may reveal that true rigor then develops as the cellular chemical processes recommence.

In temperate conditions rigor can be first detected in the face between 1 and 4 hours and in the limbs between 4 and 6 hours after death, and the strength of the rigor increases for the next 6–12 hours. Once established, rigor will remain static until decomposition of the cellular contents begins and the muscle cells lose their cohesion. The secondary flaccidity becomes apparent from 24 to 50 hours after death.

It is best to test for rigor across a joint using very gentle pressure from one or two fingers only; the aim is to detect the presence and extent of the stiffness, not to 'break' it. If rigor is broken by applying too much force, those muscle groups cannot reliably be tested again.

A crude but useful aide-memoire is:

Body feels warm and flaccid – dead less than 3 hours.
Body feels warm and stiff – dead 3–8 hours.
Body feels cold and stiff – dead 8–36 hours.
Body feels cold and flaccid – dead more than 36 hours.

CADAVERIC RIGIDITY

This is a forensic rarity that is always quoted in textbooks – and in court when rigor is being discussed! Cadaveric rigidity is the stiffness of muscles that is said to have its onset immediately at death, and the basis

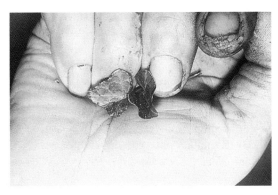

Figure 6.1 Cadaveric rigidity – a rare condition. This victim grasped at some ivy as he fell into water.

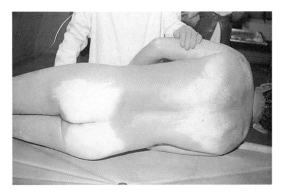

Figure 6.2 Normal distribution of post-mortem hypostasis in a body which lay on its back after death. The white areas are due to pressure upon the ground.

for this concept is the finding of items gripped firmly in the hand of the deceased before the onset of normal rigor. Most cases are said to be related to individuals who are at high levels of emotional or physical stress immediately before death and many reports relate to battlefield casualties, but there are many reports of individuals recovered from rivers with weeds or twigs grasped firmly in their hand or the finger of a suicidal shooting found tightly gripping the trigger. It is suggested that the mechanism for this phenomenon is possibly neurogenic, but no scientifically satisfactory explanation has been given. It is clearly not the same chemical process as true rigor and it is better that the term 'instantaneous rigor' is no longer used.

POST-MORTEM HYPOSTASIS

Cessation of the circulation and the relaxation of the muscular tone of the vascular bed allow simple fluid movement to occur within the blood vessels. Theoretically, currents will occur between warmer and colder areas of the body and this may be of importance in the redistribution of drugs and chemicals after death. There is also the filling of the dependent blood vessels.

The passive settling of red blood cells under the influence of gravity to the blood vessels in lowest areas of the body is important forensically. It produces a pink or bluish colour to these lowest areas and it is this colour change that is called post-mortem hypostasis. This same change has also been called post-mortem lividity and also suggillation. Hypostasis is not always seen in a body and it may be absent in the young, the

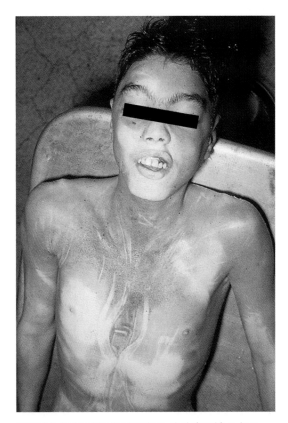

Figure 6.3 Post-mortem hypostasis on a body found face down on a bed. The linear marks are formed by pressure from creases in the blanket. The pale areas around the mouth and nose are not necessarily signs of suffocation.

old and the clinically anaemic or in those who have died from severe blood loss. It may be masked by dark skin colours, by jaundice or by some dermatological conditions.

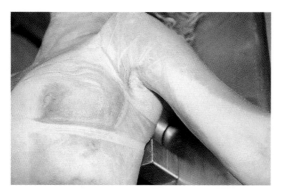

Figure 6.4 Hypostasis affected by simple pressure on the skin from tight clothing – here the marks of the cup and strap of a bra are easily seen on the chest. The pallor of the arm is due to flexion of the elbow with the forearm pressing against the upper arm.

As most bodies fall down or lie horizontally when dead and most are placed in a supine position, hypostasis commonly forms on the back, buttocks, thighs, calves and the back of the neck. However, hypostasis occurs only where the superficial blood vessels can be distended by blood and, if the body is lying on a firm surface, the weight of the body will compress those areas of the skin that are in contact with the surface and prevent the filling of the blood vessels. These compressed areas will remain pale and their pallor will be all the more striking because of the surrounding hypostasis. This is commonly referred to as blanching. Blanching may also be caused by pressure of clothing or by contact of one area of the body with another, in which case 'mirror image' blanching may be seen.

If a body has lain face downwards, the blanching around the mouth may be striking and may lead to a suggestion of asphyxiation, particularly suffocation. This problem may be compounded in congestive deaths in which petechial haemorrhages of the face are also found. It is imperative that any diagnosis of asphyxiation is confirmed by the presence of other pathological features such as bruising to the face, lips or gums and such a diagnosis should not be based on these pale areas alone.

The site and distribution of the hypostasis must be considered in the light of the position of the body after death. A body left suspended after hanging will develop deep hypostasis of the lower legs and arms, with none visible on the torso, whereas a body that has partially fallen head first out of bed will have the most prominent hypostatic changes of the head and upper chest.

The colour of hypostasis is variable and may extend from pink to dark pink to deep purple and, in some congestive hypoxic states, to blue. In general, no attempt should be made to form any conclusions about the cause of death from these variations of colour, but there are, however, a few colour changes that may act as indicators of possible causes of death: the cherry pink colour of carbon monoxide poisoning, the dark red or brick red colour associated with cyanide poisoning, and infection by *Clostridium perfringens*, which is said to result in bronze hypostasis.

The hypostatic changes associated with hypothermia deserve special mention because they are unusual. The colour of hypostasis can be unusually pink and it has a prominent distribution around the large joints as well as over the dependent areas of the body. However, any body simply stored in a refrigerator will often develop the same colour of hypostasis but the distribution will not be the same.

The time taken for hypostasis to appear is so variable that it has no significant role in determining the time of death. Movement of a body will have an effect on hypostasis, as the red blood cells continue to move under the influence of gravity. Even after the normal post-mortem coagulation of the blood has occurred, movement of the red blood cells, although severely reduced, still continues.

This continued ability of the red blood cells to move is important because changes in the position of a body after the initial development of hypostasis will result in redistribution of the hypostasis and examination of the body may reveal two overlapping patterns.

COOLING OF THE BODY AFTER DEATH

On one hand, the cooling of the body after death can be viewed as a simple physical property of a warm object in a cooler environment. Newton's Law of Cooling states that heat will pass from the warmer body to the cooler environment and the temperature of the body will fall. However, a body is not a uniform structure: its temperature will not fall evenly and because each body will lie in its own unique environment, each body will cool at a different speed, depending upon the many factors surrounding it. Much research has been done on this and it is well reviewed in the book *Estimation of the Time Since Death* (see 'Recommended reading').

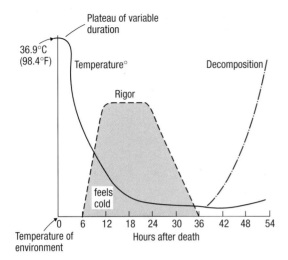

Figure 6.5 The sequence of major changes after death in a temperate environment. Note that the core body temperature does not show a fall for the first hour or so.

In order to use body temperature as an indicator of the time of death, we must make three basic forensic assumptions.

1 The first forensic assumption is that the body temperature was 37°C at the time of death. However, humans are very variable and their temperature will vary during the day (diurnal variation) and will also be altered by exercise, by illness, in women of reproductive age by the stage of the menstrual cycle and by a host of other factors.

2 The second forensic assumption is that it is possible to take one, or maybe a few, temperature readings and extrapolate a temperature to apply to this non-uniform body as a whole. Clearly, the more readings that are taken, the more likely it is that the mathematical formulae will be useful.

3 The third forensic assumption is that the body has lain in a thermally static environment so that this complex cooling is not further complicated by changes in the environment. Unfortunately, this is not the case and even bodies lying in a confined domestic environment may be subject to the daily variations of the central heating system, while the variations imposed on a body lying outside are potentially so great that no sensible 'average' can be achieved.

Other variables and factors also affect the rate of cooling of a body (listed below) and together they show why the sensible forensic pathologist will be reluctant to make any pronouncement on the time of death based on the body temperature alone.

- Mass of the body.
- Mass/surface area.
- Body temperature at the time of death.
- Site of reading of body temperature(s).
- Posture of the body – extended or curled into a fetal position.
- Clothing – type of material, position on the body – or lack of it.
- Obesity – because fat is a good insulator.
- Emaciation – lack of muscle bulk allows a body to cool faster.
- Environmental temperature.
- Winds, draughts, rain, humidity etc.

Despite all of these problems, the pathologist may still be asked by the police or by the court for an estimate of the time of death. There would appear to be two forms of this question. The simpler question asks the pathologist to consider whether the time of death given by a witness is, or is not, consistent with the pathological findings. The second form of the question is the wider one, commonly asked in the absence of any other evidence, and it is for an estimate of the time of death based on the pathological findings alone. Great care must be taken in answering both questions, and the reliability or otherwise of the opinion must be stated.

ESTIMATION OF THE TIME OF DEATH

Of the three historic pathological features that were used to estimate death, only the fall in body temperature has withstood the test of science; the others – rigor mortis and hypostasis – have now been shown to be utterly unreliable and will not be considered further.

Body temperature

Traditionally, the temperature of the body was taken rectally using a long, low-reading thermometer (0–50°C was considered to be adequate). However, there are problems with using this site because any interference with the anus or rectum before a full forensic examination of the area in a good light may

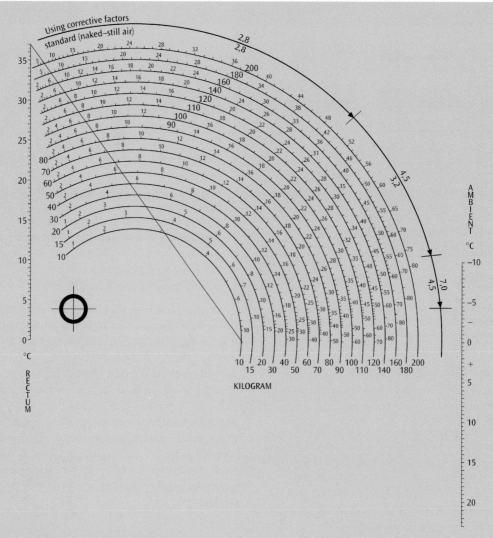

The temperature–time of death relating nomogram (for ambient temperatures up to 25°C). Permissible variation of 95% (±h). The nomogram expresses the death-time (t) by:

$$\frac{T_{rectum} - T_{ambient}}{37.2 - T_{ambient}} = 1.25 \exp(Bt) - .25 \exp(5Bt); \quad B = -1.2815 (kg^{-.625}) + .0284$$

The nomogram is related to the chosen standard; that is, naked body extended lying in still air. Cooling conditions differing from the chosen standard may be proportionally adjusted by corrective factors of the real body weight, giving the corrected body weight by which the death-time is to be read off. Factors above 1.0 may correct thermal isolation conditions, and factors below 1.0 may correct conditions accelerating the heat loss of a body.

How to read off the time of death

1 Connect the points of the scales by a straight line according to the rectal and the ambient temperature. It crosses the diagonal of the nomogram at a special point.

2 Draw a second straight line going through the centre of the circle, below left of nomogram, and the intersection of the first line and the diagonal. The second line crosses the semi-circle of the body weight: the time of death can be read off. The second line touches a segment of the outermost semi-circle. Here can be seen the permissible variation of 95%.

Example: temperature of the rectum 26.4°C; ambient temperature 12°C; body weight 90 kg.

Result: time of death 16 ± 1.8 hours. Statement: the death occurred within 13.2 and 18.8 (13 and 19)

Empiric corrective factors of the body weight

Dry clothing/covering	In air	Corrective factor	Wet through clothing/ covering wet body surface	In air/water
		3.5	naked	flowing
		.5	naked	still
		.7	naked	moving
		.7	1–2 thin layers	moving
naked	moving	.75		
1–2 thin layers	moving	.9	2 or more thicker	moving
naked	still	1.0		
1–2 thin layers	still	1.1	2 thicker layers	still
2–3 thin layers		1.2	more than 2 thicker layers	still
1–2 thicker layers	moving or still	1.2		
3–4 thin layers		1.3		
more thin/thicker layers	without influence	1.45		
thick bedspread + clothing		1.8		
combined		2.4		

hours before the time of measurement (with a reliability of 95%).

Note: If the values of the ambient temperature and/or the body weight (see 'corrective factors') are called into question, repeat the procedure with other values which might be possible. The range of death-time can be seen in this way.

Requirements for the use

- No strong radiation (e.g. sun, heater, cooling system).
- No strong fever or general hypothermia.
- No uncertain (+) severe changes of the cooling conditions during the period between the time of death and examination (e.g. the place of death must be the same as where the body was found).
- No high thermal conductivity of the surface beneath the body (++).

+ Known changes can be taken into account: a change of the ambient temperature can often be evaluated (e.g. contact the weather station); use the mean ambient temperature of the period in question. Changes by the operations of the investigators (e.g. take any cover off) since finding the body are negligible: take the conditions before into account!

++ Measure the temperature of the surface beneath the body too. If there is a significant difference between the temperature of the air and the surface temperature, use the mean.

Note: for the selection of the corrective factor of any case, only the clothing or covering of the *lower trunk* is relevant! Personal experience is needed, nevertheless this is quickly achieved by the consistent use of the method.

Marshall, T.K., Hoare, F.E. 1962: Estimating the Time of Death. *J Forensic Sci* **7**, 56–81, 189–210, 211–12.

Henssge, D. 1979: Precision of Estimating the Time of Death by Mathematical Expression of Rectal Body Cooling. *Z Rechtsmed* **83**, 49–67.

Henssge, C. 1981: Estimation of Death-Time by Computing the Rectal Body Cooling Under Various Cooling Conditions. *Z Rechtsmed* **87**, 147–8.

Henssge, C., Brinkmann, B., Püschel, K. 1984: Determination of Time of Death by Measuring the Rectal Temperature in Corpses Suspended in Water. *Z Rechtsmed* **92**, 255–76.

confuse or contaminate later investigations into the presence of semen, blood, hairs etc.

The development of small electronic temperature probes with rapid response times and digital readouts has revolutionized the taking of body temperatures.

These probes have allowed the use of other orifices, including the nose and ear, although it must be remembered that these areas are unlikely to register the same temperature as the deep rectum or the liver.

Currently, the most useful method of estimating the time of death is Henssge's Nomogram (which is explained in some detail on the preceeding pages). Crucially, the 95 per cent accuracy claimed for this method is, at best, only 2.8 hours on either side of the most likely time – a total spread of over 5.5 hours. Henssge's Normogram relies on three measurements – body temperature, ambient temperature and body weight – and lack of accuracy in any one of these will degrade the final result. In addition, there is the application of empirical corrective factors to allow for clothing, air movement and/or water and it should be noted that application of these empirical factors can significantly lengthen the time spans that lie within the 95 per cent confidence limits.

The need to record the ambient temperature poses some problems because pathologists are seldom in a position to do this at the time of discovery and, as their arrival at the scene is often delayed by some tens of minutes or hours, it is most unlikely that the temperature at that time will still be of relevance. Therefore, the first police officers or scientists at the scene should be encouraged to take the ambient temperature adjacent to the body and to record the time that they made their measurement. An alteration of 5°C in the ambient temperature may lead to, at least, a 1-hour alteration in the most likely time of death.

Many pathologists have in the past used various 'rules of thumb' to calculate the time of death from the body temperature but these are, overall, so unreliable that they should not now be used.

Sometimes the perceived warmth of the body to touch is mentioned in court as an indicator of the time of death; this assessment is so unreliable as to be useless and is even more so if the pathologist is asked to comment upon the reported perceptions of another person. If the pathologists themselves have made the observation, it has slightly more validity and, in conjunction with a proper assessment of rigor, may be applied in the broad framework of the aide-memoire noted earlier.

Other methods of estimating the time of death

Various other methods have been researched in a vain attempt to find the hands of the post-mortem clock. Biochemical methods, including vitreous humor potassium levels and changes in enzyme and electrolyte levels elsewhere in the body, have been researched; some remain as interesting research tools but none has been successful in routine work.

Examination of gastric contents may confirm the constituents of the final meal but it will not determine how long before death the meal was eaten. Gastric emptying has been completely discredited as a means of estimating the time of death because there is great individual variation even in normal conditions and digestion of food and gastric emptying may cease if the individual is under physical or emotional stress.

Of considerably more value is the work of the forensic entomologist, who can determine a probable time of death – in the region of days to months – from examination of the populations and stages of development of the various insects that invade a body. Initially, the sarcophagous flies – the bluebottle (*Callphorae*), the greenbottle (*Lucilla*) and houseflies (*Musca*) – lay their eggs on moist areas, particularly the eyes, nose, mouth and, if exposed, the anus and genitalia. The eggs hatch into larvae, which grow and shed their skins a number of times, each moult being called an instar. Finally, they pupate and a new winged insect emerges. The time from egg laying through the instars to pupation depends on the species and on the ambient temperature, but in general it is about 21–24 days.

Other animals, both large and small, will arrive to feed on the body, the species and the rapidity of their arrival depending on the time of year and the environment. The examination of buried bodies or skeletal remains will usually require the combined specialist skills of the forensic pathologist, an anthropologist and an entomologist.

Decomposition

In the cycle of life, dead bodies are usually returned, through reduction into their various components, to the chemical pool that is the earth. Some components will do this by entering the food chain at almost any level – from ant to tiger – whereas others will be reduced to simple chemicals by the autolytic enzymic processes built into the lysosomes of each cell.

The early changes of decomposition are important because they may be confused by the police or members of the public with the signs of violence or trauma.

Putrefaction

This is by far the commonest route of decomposition taken by any body after death and this route will be followed unless some unusual conditions apply. This form of decomposition results in liquefaction of the soft tissues over a period of time. The time of visible onset and the speed with which this process proceeds are, of course, functions of the ambient temperature: the warmer the temperature, the earlier the process starts and the faster it progresses.

In temperate climates the process is usually first visible to the naked eye at about 3–4 days as an area of green discoloration of the right iliac fossa of the anterior abdominal wall. This change is the result of the extension of the commensal gut bacteria through the bowel wall and into the skin, where they decompose haemoglobin, resulting in the green colour. The right iliac fossa is the usual origin as the caecum lies close to the abdominal wall at this site. This green colour is but an external mark of the profound changes that are occurring in the body as the gut bacteria move out of the bowel lumen into the abdominal cavity and the blood vessels.

The blood vessels provide an excellent channel through which the bacteria can spread with some ease throughout the body. Their passage is marked by the decomposition of haemoglobin which, when present in the superficial vessels, results in linear branching patterns of brown discoloration of the skin that is called 'marbling'. The colour changes gradually affect most of the skin and, as the superficial layers of the skin lose cohesions, blisters full of red or brown fluid form in many areas. When the blisters burst, the skin sloughs off.

Considerable gas formation is common and the body begins to swell, with bloating of the face, abdomen, breasts and genitals. The increased internal pressure causes the eyes and tongue to protrude and forces bloody fluid up from the lungs and it will often leak out of the mouth and nose as 'purge'.

The role of flies and maggots and other animals is discussed above; domestic animals are not excluded from this process.

The exact time scale for this process cannot be predicted, as the vagaries of the ambient temperature and many other aspects of the environment generally and the microenvironment specifically may have significant effects to either extend or shorten the process.

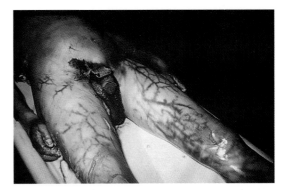

Figure 6.6 Early decomposition showing marbling of skin due to bacterial growth spreading through the venous system.

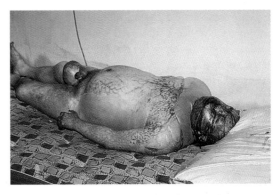

Figure 6.7 Putrefaction after about a week in temperate summer conditions. The skin is discoloured and there is gaseous distension of the face, abdomen and scrotum.

However, in general terms, within a week or so the body cavities will burst and the tissues will liquefy and drain away into the underlying ground. The prostate and the uterus are relatively resistant to putrefaction and they may survive for months, as may the tendons and ligaments. Eventually, skeletalization will be complete and unless the bones are destroyed by larger animals, they may remain for years.

Mummification

A body lying in dry conditions, either climatic or in the microenvironment, may desiccate instead of putrefying – a process known as mummification. Mummified tissue is dry and leathery and often brown in colour. It is most commonly seen in warm or hot environments such as the dessert and led to the spontaneous mummification of bodies buried in the sand in Egypt. However, it is not only bodies from hot dry climates that can be mummified, as the micro-environment necessary for mummification may exist anywhere.

Mummification of newborn infants whose bodies are placed in cool dry environments, (e.g. below the floor boards) is common, but adults too can be mummified if they lie in dry places, preferably with a draught. Mummification is, however, much more likely in the thin individual whose body will cool and desiccate quickly.

Mummification need not affect the whole body, and some parts may show the normal putrefactive decomposition, skeletalization or formation of adipocere, depending on the conditions. Mummified tissues are not immune to degradation and invasion by rodents, beetles and moths, especially the Brown House Moth, in temperate climates.

Adipocere

Adipocere is a chemical change in the body fat, which is hydrolysed to a waxy compound not unlike soap. The need for water means that this process is most commonly seen in bodies found in wet conditions (i.e. submerged in water or buried in wet ground) but this is not always the case and some bodies from dry vaults have been found to have adipocere formation, presumably the original body water being sufficient to allow for the hydrolysis of the fat.

In the early stages of formation, adipocere is a pale, rancid, greasy semi-fluid material with a most unpleasant smell. As the hydrolysis progresses, the material becomes more brittle and whiter and, when fully formed, adipocere is a grey, firm, waxy compound which maintains the shape of the body. The speed with which adipocere can develop is variable; it would usually be expected to take weeks or months, but it is reported to have occurred in as little as 3 weeks. All three stages of adipocere formation can co-exist and they can also be found with areas of mummification and putrefaction if the conditions are correct.

Immersion and burial

Immersion in water or burial will slow the process of decomposition. It is said that a body in air will decompose twice as fast as a body in water and four times as fast as a body under the ground.

Water temperatures are usually lower than those on land. A body in water may adopt a number of positions, but the most common in the early stage is with

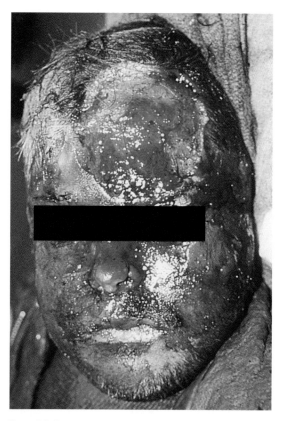

Figure 6.9 Post-mortem damage to a body found on a river bank that was probably caused by rodents.

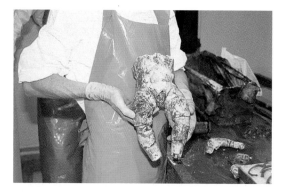

Figure 6.8 Adipocere formation in an infant buried for 3 years. The body fat has been converted into brittle waxy material, which forms a shell around the skeleton.

the air-containing chest floating uppermost and the head and limbs hanging downwards. Hypostasis follows the usual pattern and affects the head and limbs, and these areas may also be damaged by contact with the bottom if the water is shallow.

The first change that affects the body in water is the loss of epidermis. Gaseous decomposition progresses and the bloated body is often, but not always, lifted to the surface by these gases, most commonly at about 1 week but this time is extremely variable. Marine predators will replace the animals found on land and they can cause extensive damage. The exposure to water can, in some cases, predispose to the formation of adipocere, but this is unusual unless a body lies underwater for many weeks.

Burial

The effects and the time scale of the changes following burial are so variable that little specific can be said other than buried bodies generally decay more slowly, especially if they are buried deep within the ground. The level of moisture in the surrounding soil and acidity of the soil will both significantly alter the speed of decomposition.

Skeletalization

The speed of skeletalization will depend on many factors, including the climate and the microenvironment around the body. It will occur much more quickly in a body on the surface of the ground than in one that is buried. Generally speaking, in a formally buried body, the soft tissues will be absent by 2 years. Tendons, ligaments hair and nails will be identifiable for some time after that.

At about 5 years, the bones will be bare and disarticulated, although fragments of articular cartilage may be identified for many years and for several years the bones will feel slightly greasy and, if cut with a saw, a wisp of smoke and a smell of burning organic material may be present. Examination of the bone marrow space may reveal residual organic material that can sometimes be suitable for specialist DNA analysis.

Dating bones, as with all post-mortem dating, is fraught with difficulty. The microenvironment in which the bone has lain is of crucial importance and

the examination and dating of bones are now a specialist subject and, if in doubt, the forensic pathologist should enlist the assistance of anthropologists or archaeologists who have the specialist skills and techniques to manage this type of material.

In the UK, the medico-legal interest in bones fades rapidly if a bone has been dead for more than 70–80 years, because even if it was from a criminal death, it is most unlikely that the killer would still be alive. Carbon-14 dating is of no use in this short time scale, but examination of the bones for levels of strontium-90, which was released into the atmosphere in high levels only after the detonation of the nuclear bombs in the 1940s, allows for the differentiation of bones from before and after that time.

Post-mortem injuries

Dead bodies are not immune to injuries and can be exposed to a wide range of trauma and it is important to bear this possibility in mind when examining any body so that these injuries are not confused with injuries sustained during life.

The injuries may be caused during an initial collapse and these will usually comprise areas of laceration to the head and scalp, which can be extremely hard to interpret. Predation by land animals and insects has been mentioned earlier and can cause serious damage to the body: if there is any doubt about bite marks, an odontologist should be consulted. In water, fish, crustaceans and larger animals can also cause severe damage, but there is the added damage caused by the water logging of the skin and the movement of the body across the bottom or against the

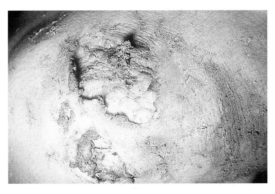

Figure 6.10 Post-mortem injury to the knee, with no evidence of bleeding or reddening of the margins of the laceration.

banks. Contact with boats and propellers will generally lead to patterned injuries that should be easily recognizable.

It is not true to say that post-mortem injuries do not bleed because many do leak blood, especially those on the scalp and in bodies recovered from water. The confirmation that a wound is post mortem in origin may be extremely difficult because injuries inflicted in the last few minutes of life and those that were caused after death may appear exactly the same. In general, post-mortem injuries do not have a rim of an early inflammatory response in the wound edges, but the lack of this response does not exclude an injury inflicted in the last moments of life.

Chapter seven

Identification of the Living and the Dead

There are numerous medico-legal reasons why it is important to be able to establish the identity of a living individual or of a dead body. The living may not be able to identify themselves for a variety of reasons: coma, amnesia, infancy or mental defect and possibly even severe language barriers may prevent people from giving information about themselves. Alternatively, an individual may simply chose to conceal his true identity by providing false information. Even if the identity of the individual is known, other personal details, for instance their exact age, may need to be confirmed for the purposes of immigration or inheritance.

The identity of a corpse is of paramount importance in the investigation of any death and forms the first part of a coroner's inquisition. Where the body is decomposed or skeletalized, it will not be possible to obtain visual identification and so identification can be more difficult. In some homicides the body may be so injured that visual identification is not reliable or it may have been deliberately mutilated or concealed until post-mortem changes make visual recognition impossible. Mass disasters, either natural such as earthquakes or man-made such as air crashes, also require the identification of the dead.

The detailed examination of the dead for evidence of identity is a specialized task for the forensic pathologist, forensic odontologist, anthropologist and other experts, but every doctor should have some idea of the features that can be used to establish the identity of a person, dead or alive.

MORPHOLOGICAL CHARACTERISTICS

Identity cannot be established by the simple measurement of a set of parameters of an individual or a body. It can only be established by matching the parameters that can be measured or seen on an individual with the same parameters that were known to apply to or to be present on a named individual. Identification is established by matching an array of general observations made about the body to an array of general information known to be true about that particular individual. The finding of a specific feature, or a combination of specific features, that is known to be possessed by that individual alone will add considerable weight to the conclusions.

In both the living and dead, the height, weight and general physique need to be recorded and compared. Hair colour and length, including beaching or dying, the presence of a beard or moustache, the amount and distribution of other body hair, including sites that are commonly shaved, all need to be established. Skin pigmentation, racial and ethnic facial appearances, such as flared nostrils, epicanthic folds etc., are also obvious features which need to recorded in a standard fashion. Eye colour is useful in the Caucasian race but of little use in the negroid and mongoloid races, virtually all of whom have brown irises. However, caution must be used for the dead Caucasian as post-mortem changes tend to darken blue or green eyes so that, within a day or so of death, they appear brownish.

All clothing, jewellery and other ornaments on the person must be recorded and photographed as they may provide useful information about the sex, race and even occupation and social status of the body, even if they are not sufficient for identification. Tattoos, surgical scars, old injuries, congenital deformities, striae from childbirth, tribal scars or markings, circumcision, moles, warts and other skin blemishes etc. must be carefully recorded and, if unusual, photographed because a relative, friend or doctor may be able to confirm an identity from these features.

In a living person or an intact body, the facial appearance is all important, both from racial aspects and from individual appearances. Frontal and profile photographs should be taken for comparison.

The age of living people or of bodies can be assessed on general appearance, such as grey or white hair, an arcus senilis around the iris of the eye, and loss of elasticity (wrinkling) of the skin. Senile hyperkeratosis and moles, red Campbell de Morgan spots and arthritic changes are also general indicators of advanced age. In the young, tooth eruption is important and also relatively accurate.

Ossification centres and epiphyseal union can be examined by x-ray or visualized in the dead. The risks of exposure to x-rays will need to be balanced against the benefit to be gained from the radiological information and this type of examination should not be undertaken lightly. Fortunately, other scanning techniques, including magnetic resonance imaging (MRI), which are not associated with long-term risks can now be used with safety.

FINGERPRINTS

These are mainly a matter for the police, but the doctor may be asked to assist in obtaining them. The recovery of the fingerprints from decomposing and damaged bodies requires the use of specialized techniques which are the province of the fingerprint expert. Prints may often be obtained from desquamated skin or from the underlying epidermis after shedding of the stratum corneum following prolonged submersion.

The pattern of the fingerprint comprises arches, loops (which open towards the radial or ulnar side),

whorls or combinations of those three patterns, but as important as these patterns is the position of minute defects on the ridges. It is traditional to require no less than 16 points of similarity before declaring prints to be identical. It has been calculated that the chances of there being an identical fingerprint in two persons is about one in 64 billion. Such a match would be an entirely random event because even identical twins do not have identical fingerprints.

In addition to fingerprints, palm and sole prints are identifiable and research is also being carried out on lip crease patterns, ear shape and the vein pattern on the dorsum of the hands, all of which seem to have individual characteristics, but no statistically reliable basis for any identification has yet been established.

IDENTITY FROM TEETH

Forensic odontology (forensic dentistry) is now a forensic specialty in its own right and, wherever possible, medico-legal problems involving teeth or bite marks should be passed to a dentist who has been trained and is qualified in forensic work. The forensic odontologist has two main areas of expertise: assisting in identification, usually of the dead, and the examination and comparison of bite marks. (Bite marks are discussed in detail in Chapter 9.) In the living, odontology can also be used in the estimation of age in young people, especially for purposes of immigration, adoption and similar civil matters.

The forensic odontologist is commonly requested to confirm the identity of a body by comparing antemortem dental chartings with the information gained from a direct examination of the teeth. The odontologist may also be asked to make dental chartings of bodies whose identity remains unknown or unconfirmed despite a police investigation, so that, should dental information become available at a later date, the two sets of records may be then be compared. It is important to remember that neither a living individual person nor a body can be identified simply by taking a dental chart – that chart has to be compared with, and found to match, a chart whose origins are known.

The forensic odontologist is of prime importance in mass disasters where trauma is likely to make visual identification impossible. The great advantage of dental identification is that the teeth are the hardest and most resistant tissues in the body and can survive total decomposition and even severe fire, short of actual cremation.

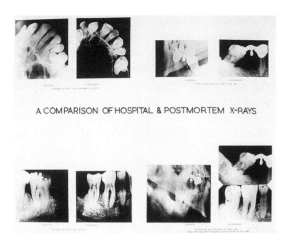

Figure 7.1 The use of comparison of ante-mortem and post-mortem dental x-rays to confirm an identity.

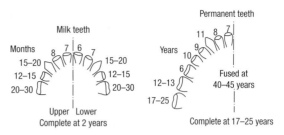

Figure 7.2 Identification of the stage of eruption of teeth can provide useful information about the age of the individual up to about 20–25 years.

Where no forensic odontologist is available, a doctor may be able to seek the help of a clinical dentist in charting the teeth and comparing the results with any available records. If necessary, these charts may be forwarded to a forensic odontologist almost anywhere in the world for an urgent opinion using fax or the Internet. If the doctor has to work alone, he should use a standard dental chart to record all the features he can find, which can be supported by photographs if necessary.

Where no previous records are available, examination of the mouth and the teeth can still give some general information on age, sex and ethnic origin.

- In a young person aged 20–25 years or less, the eruption of the deciduous and permanent teeth can be compared with standard charts, but care must be taken not to expect too much accuracy as it is reported that in girls and in hot countries tooth eruption may be up to a year earlier than normally expected. Tooth loss is much less predictable and a very wide age range exists as some people may lose their teeth early because of disease. In the absence of teeth, a general idea of age can also be gained by the appearance of the jaws, especially the mandible, as the edentulous jaw is thinner.

  There are sophisticated methods of determining personal age from teeth, Gustafson's technique, using thin ground sections, and an evaluation of attrition (wearing) on the occlusal surfaces being two examples, but these techniques are only for the expert odontologist.

- In the hands of an expert, the teeth may also give a clue as to sex and race. The former is not very reliable and depends upon size and molar cusp numbers, the identification of ethnicity being limited to the upper incisors, which in some mongoloid races show a characteristic 'shovel-shaped' concavity, and the palate in negroid people is said to have a deeper U-shape.

IDENTIFICATION OF THE ORIGIN OF TISSUE OR SAMPLES

This is important for several reasons:

- to show whether blood, semen, saliva or other stains on bodies, weapons, clothing or elsewhere could, or could not, have come from a particular suspect or victim;
- to match fragmented human remains in air and other disasters or in mutilating homicides;
- to resolve paternity, maternity and inheritance disputes.

THE INDIVIDUALITY OF CELLS

Historically it was the ABO blood groups, first identified by Landsteiner in 1900, that allowed the identification of some individuality of this one type of cell. Since then, many other blood group systems, which characterize blood in many different ways, have been discovered and of these systems including the Rhesus (Rh), Kell, Duffy and Lewis groups together with other features such as protein complexes, haptoglobins and the blood enzyme systems such as phosphoglucomutase. By combining these tests it was possible to exclude approximately 93 per cent of non-matching samples but they could never positively identify the sample (Table 7.1).

Table 7.1 Percentage Chance of Exclusion by Individual Systems

	Percentage exclusion
Red cell antigens	
MNSs	32.1
Rh	28.0
ABO	17.6
Duffy	4.8
Kidd	4.5
Kell	3.3
Luthran	3.3
Serum proteins	
Haptoglobin (Hp)	17.5
Gc	14.5
C3	14.2
Gm	6.5
Red cell enzymes	
Erythrocyte acid phosphatase (EAP)	21.0
Glutamate pyruvate transaminase (GPT)	19.0
Glycoxalase (Glo)	18.4
Phosphoglucomutase (PGM)	14.5
Esterase D (EsD)	9.0
Adenylate kinase (AK)	4.5
Adenosine deaminase (ADA)	4.5
6-Phosphogluconate dehydrogenase (6-GPD)	2.5
Total combined chance using all systems	93.0

This bank of tests was used for the forensic identification of blood and other body fluids but has now been replaced by DNA analysis of human tissue and fluid, which is claimed to be nearly 100 per cent accurate, both in exclusion and in identification.

IDENTIFICATION BY DNA PROFILING

Following the discoveries of Sir Alec Jeffreys, a British geneticist, this powerful new tool has radically altered forensic investigations. The specificity of deoxyribonucleic acid (DNA) profiles is so great in statistical terms that it can be reliably specific to any individual.

The molecule of DNA has two strands of sugar and phosphate molecules that are linked by combinations of four bases – adenine, thymine, cytosine and guanine – forming the double helix of DNA. Only about 10 per cent of the molecule is used for genetic coding (the active genes), the remainder being 'silent'. In these silent zones, there are between 200 and 14 000 repeats of identical sequences of the four bases. Jeffreys found that adjacent sequences were constant for a given individual and that they were transmitted, like blood groups, from the DNA of each parent. Only uni-ovular twins have the same sequences; otherwise, the chances of two unrelated individuals sharing the same sequence is one in a billion or higher. The statistical analysis of DNA identification is extremely complex and it is important that any calculations are based upon the DNA characteristics of a relevant population and not upon the characteristics of a 'standard' population somewhere else in the world.

The technique of determining the sequences is extremely complex, relying on cutting the DNA strands at predetermined points by the use of restriction enzymes. The fragments of DNA are separated using electrophoresis and the different fragments are then identified using a radioactive probe. Autoradiography produces a picture of a series of bars of varying density and spacing, which bears a marked resemblance to the 'bar code' used for pricing articles in a supermarket. From the presence of different bars in given positions, comparisons may be made with other samples, known or unknown – the classical forensic 'comparison technique'.

Crucially, there is now no need to match blood with blood and semen with semen, as all the DNA in one individual's body must of necessity be identical. A perpetrator leaving any of his cells or body fluids at a scene is leaving proof of his presence.

Contamination

As the scientists become more and more proficient at extracting and amplifying smaller and smaller amounts of genetic material, so the risks of contamination increase. Scene examination must now be approached with great care and with sufficient protective clothing to prevent the investigators obscuring any relevant DNA by their own material inadvertently shed from exposed skin, sneezing etc. There is now the need for investigators to provide exclusion DNA samples in the same way as fingerprints were once provided.

Paternity/maternity testing

Another medico-legal use for DNA is in paternity testing, in which, for the first time, a positive identity can be made rather than relying on the exclusions possible with blood group methods. Every bar in the 'bar code' must have come from either the father or mother, half from each. In testing, the coding is made from the mother, the child and the putative father. The bars in the child's profile are first matched with the mother's, so the remaining bars must all have come from the father and complete matching of the bars confirms paternity, whereas any discrepancy will exclude it. Occasionally, similar testing must be performed to establish who the parents are following disputes in maternity units.

Samples required for DNA analysis

Samples suitable for DNA analysis are derived from any nucleated cellular material such as white blood cells, hair root bulb cells, spermatozoa etc. Initially, relatively large samples were required for this analysis, but the development of the polymerase chain reaction (PCR), which can 'grow up' or 'amplify' small amounts of DNA, means that positive DNA identification can be made from the smallest of samples.

When taking samples either at post mortem or from a living victim or from the accused, there is seldom any problem with the size of the sample that can be taken. Samples from areas of staining of the scene, the deceased, the living victim or the accused may pose different problems as these may be very small areas of blood, semen staining etc., and these samples must be collected with great care to ensure that contamination is kept to a minimum.

Blood and hair with roots are used in the living and the dead, samples of spleen can be taken at post mortem and buccal smears can be taken from the living. If there is the possibility of a sexual assault, or perhaps in all cases of suspicious death, vaginal, anal and penile swabs should be taken. If there is to be any delay in getting samples to the laboratory, they should be frozen solid at −20°C or as instructed by the laboratory.

TATTOOS AND BODY PIERCING

The main use of tattoos in forensic medicine is in the identification of the bodies of unknown persons. Once again, the simple presence of a tattoo does not constitute identification and there has to be a comparison with the tattoos of a known individual. Photographs

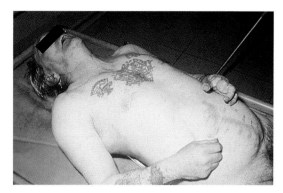

Figure 7.3 The identification of this body was considerably assisted by the tattoos, the surgical scar and the absence of two fingers.

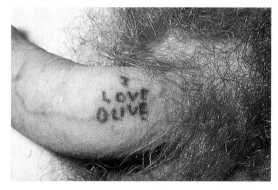

Figure 7.4 This unusual tattoo aided identification of this body.

should be taken or drawings made which can be used if a visual identification is not possible or so that they can be circulated when the identity is not known.

There is a huge diversity of skin tattoos in Western society, some of which may have specific meaning or significance within certain subgroups of society, but there is also much 'folklore' about the significance of tattoos, a large amount of which is fiction. Names within tattoos may be useful but, as partners may change rapidly, they may be of little value. It is said that girls more often have their boyfriend's name tattooed than vice versa. Tattoos inside the lips, such as the number 13, may still identify a drug dealer but are more likely to indicate time in prison. Tattoos from the concentration camps and ghettos of the Second World War are still occasionally seen.

Decomposing bodies should be examined carefully for tattoos, which may be rendered more visible when the superficial desquamated stratum corneum is removed.

Body piercing has gained fashionable status in the West, and the site and type of piercing should be noted and the rings (as with any other jewellery) can be used as part of visual identification or can be recovered for identification by relatives if visual identification is not possible.

IDENTITY OF DECOMPOSED OR SKELETALIZED REMAINS

This is usually the task of the forensic pathologist, now most commonly with the aid of an anthropologist and other specialists if necessary. The examining doctor has to carefully document his findings with drawings and, if possible, with photographs. Wherever possible, the remains, or at least certain key parts, should be retained for later examination by experts.

When presumed skeletal remains are discovered, the investigators wish to know:

- Are the remains actually bones? Sometimes stones or even pieces of wood are mistaken by the public or police for bones: the anatomical shape and texture should be obvious to a doctor.
- Are the remains human? A doctor should be able to identify most intact long bones and a forensic pathologist almost all of the human skeleton, although phalanges, carpal and tarsal bones can be extremely difficult to positively identify as human because some animals, such as the bear, have paw bones almost identical to the human hand. It may be extremely difficult to identify fragmented bones, and the greater skills and experience of an experienced anthropologist or anatomist are invaluable. Cremated bones pose particular difficulties and these should only be examined by specialists.
- Am I dealing with one or more bodies? This question can be answered very simply if there are two skulls or two left femurs. However, if there are no obvious duplications, it is important to examine each bone carefully to assess whether the sizes and appearances match. It can be extremely difficult to exclude the possibility of co-mingling of skeletal remains, and expert anthropological advice should be sought if there is any doubt.
- What sex are the bones? The skull and the pelvis offer the best information on sexing; although the femur and sternum can provide assistance, they are of less direct value. It is important to attempt to

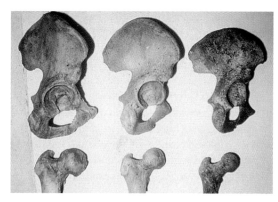

Figure 7.5 Sex differences in the pelvis and femoral head. Left to right: male, female and unknown whose characteristics are obviously female. Note also the different sizes of the femoral heads.

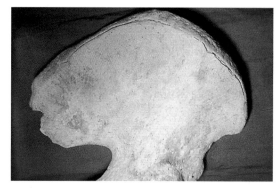

Figure 7.6 This innominate bone reveals both age and sex. The narrow greater sciatic notch is definitely male, and the clear line of the incompletely fused epiphysis at the iliac crest places the subject between 20 and 23 years of age.

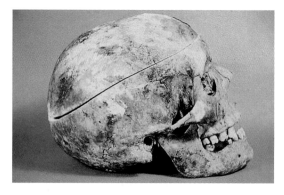

Figure 7.7 Lateral view of a skull. The forehead is vertical and there are no supraorbital ridges. The muscle attachments are not prominent and the mastoid is small – features of a female skull.

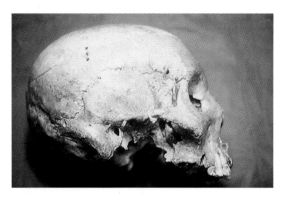

Figure 7.8 Lateral view of a skull with a sloping forehead, prominent supraorbital ridges, rough muscle attachments and a large mastoid process – features of a male skull.

determine the sex of each of these bones and not to rely on the assessment of just one. If most of the skeleton is available for examination, sexing can be carried out with over 90 per cent certainty provided that the doctor has sufficient anatomical knowledge. Specialist reference books such as *Krogman and Iscan* or the larger forensic textbooks can offer much information on all aspects of skeletal identification. However, when the issues are serious, such as in homicide, it is emphasized that expert examination by an anthropologist or anatomist is vital.

- What is the age of the person? Up to 20–25 or so, age can be estimated to within a couple of years by a combination of the eruption of the teeth and by the appearance and fusion of ossification centres and epiphyses, which can be assessed either by eye or radiologically. Epiphyseal fusion, like the eruption of the teeth, tends to be earlier in females and in tropical countries. Ageing can be more accurate in an infant or in fetal material because the rapid changes taking place at that stage of development can be used as time markers.

After about 25, ageing becomes much more difficult as all bone growth has ceased. Despite the fact that changes do still occur in the skeleton, none is of practical use. Additional data can be obtained by radiology of the trabecular pattern in the head of the humerus and femur, which re-models with age. The pubic symphysis also changes with age, but great experience is needed for its interpretation. Arthritic damage, osteoporosis and osteophytes are indicators of age, but these are extremely inexact. Specialist examination of teeth for wear and degenerative

changes can provide valuable information, but these are tests best left to an expert in the field.

- What is the height (stature) of the person? The head–heel measurement of even a completely fresh dead body is seldom the same as the person's standing height in life, due to a combination of factors, including muscle relaxation and shrinkage of intervertebral discs. If a whole skeleton is present, an approximate height can be obtained by direct measurement but, due to variable joint spaces, articular cartilage etc., this can only be, at best, an approximation. If only some bones are available, calculations can be made from the measured lengths of the femur, tibia and fibula by using a table such as that from Trotter and Gleser (Table 7.2).
- What is the race? The 'shovel-shaped' mongoloid incisor teeth have already been mentioned (page 51). There are some differences in the facial skeleton of various races, but this is very much the field of trained anthropologists and should not be attempted without their assistance.
- Can a personal identity be discovered? The previous criteria can allot bones to various groups of age, sex etc., but putting a name to the individual depends, as does all identification, upon having reliable antemortem data. Occasionally, foreign bodies such as bullets or other metallic fragments may be found embedded in the skeleton; these may either relate to the cause of death or may simply be an incidental finding. Metal prostheses are now common and may bear a unique reference number, which can sometimes be traced to an individual patient.

Where pre-mortem clinical radiographs are available, the comparison of these with the post-mortem films may give a definite identity. If a skull x-ray is available, comparison of the frontal sinus patterns is incontrovertible as no two people have the same frontal sinus outline. Expert comparisons of the lateral skull x-ray and radiographs of the upper ribs, humeri and femurs can provide useful information based partly, in the limbs, on the pattern of the cancellous bone.

FACIAL RECONSTRUCTION FROM SKULLS

In recent years, much interest has been shown in the reconstruction of the facial appearances from a bare skull. The pioneer was Gerasimov in Moscow, who measured the average soft-tissue thickness at many

Table 7.2 Stature from Bones. Trotter and Gleser's General Formulae for Reconstruction of Stature from Lengths of Dry Long Bones Without Cartilage (Constant Terms in Metric and Adapted to Imperial System)

Male White	Male African American
Stature = 63.05 + 1.31 (femur + fibula) ± 3.63 cm	Stature = 63.05 + 1.31 (femur + fibula) ± 3.63 cm
Stature = 67.09 + 1.26 (femur + tibia) ± 3.74 cm	Stature = 71.75 + 1.15 (femur + tibia) ± 3.68 cm
Stature = 75.50 + 2.60 fibula ± 3.86 cm	Stature = 72.22 + 2.10 femur ± 3.91 cm
Stature = 65.53 + 2.32 femur ± 3.95 cm	Stature = 85.36 + 2.19 tibia ± 3.96 cm
Stature = 81.93 + 2.42 tibia ± 4.00 cm	Stature = 80.07 + 2.34 fibula ± 4.02 cm
Stature = 67.97 + 1.82 (humerus + radius) ± 4.31 cm	Stature = 73.08 + 1.66 (humerus + radius) ± 4.18 cm
Stature = 66.98 + (humerus + ulna) ± 4.37 cm	Stature = 70.67 + 1.65 (humerus + ulna) ± 4.23 cm
Stature = 78.10 + 2.89 humerus ± 4.57 cm	Stature = 75.48 + 2.88 humerus ± 4.23 cm
Stature = 79.42 + 3.79 radius ± 4.66 cm	Stature = 85.43 + 3.32 radius ± 4.57 cm
Stature = 75.55 + 3.76 ulna ± 4.72 cm	Stature = 82.77 + 3.20 ulna ± 4.74 cm

Female White	Female African American
Stature = 50.12 + 0.68 humerus + 1.17 femur + 1.15 tibia ± 3.61 cm	Stature = 56.33 + 0.44 humerus − 0.20 radius + 1.46 femur + 0.86 tibia ± 3.22 cm
Stature = 53.20 + 1.39 (femur + tibia) ± 3.55 cm	Stature = 58.54 + 1.53 femur + 0.96 tibia ± 3.23 cm
Stature = 53.07 + 1.48 femur + 1.28 tibia ± 3.55 cm	Stature = 59.72 + 1.26 (femur + tibia) ± 3.28 cm
Stature = 69.61 + 2.93 fibula ± 3.57 cm	Stature = 59.76 + 2.28 femur ± 3.41 cm
Stature = 61.53 + 2.90 tibia ± 3.66 cm	Stature = 62.80 + 1.08 humerus + 1.79 tibia ± 3.58 cm
Stature = 52.77 + 1.35 humerus + 1.95 tibia ± 3.67 cm	Stature = 72.65 + 2.45 tibia ± 3.70 cm
Stature = 54.10 + 2.47 femur ± 3.72 cm	Stature = 70.90 + 2.49 fibula ± 3.80 cm
Stature = 54.93 + 4.74 radius ± 4.24 cm	Stature = 64.67 + 3.08 humerus ± 4.25 cm
Stature = 57.76 + 4.27 ulna ± 4.20 cm	Stature = 75.38 + 3.31 ulna ± 4.83 cm
Stature = 57.97 + 3.36 humerus ± 4.45 cm	Stature = 94.51 + 2.75 radius ± 5.05 cm

points on the skull and rebuilt this layer with plasticine on unknown skulls. Some research has now been performed on computerized reconstructions in which the skull is scanned into the computer and the 'tissue' is placed onto the scanned skull image electronically, with the completed image being displayed on the screen. This system has the advantage that it can be rotated electronically to obtain different views.

Whatever method is used to obtain the reconstructed face, a number of significant problems remain. One problem lies in the application of 'standard' soft-tissue thicknesses to the facial skeleton when it is the variability of the thickness of this tissue that, in part, gives individuality to a face. Another major problem is that the crucial features such as the eyes, lips and facial hair cannot be known and, as they are not dependent upon the underlying bone structure, their colour, shape, length etc. provide visual clues for identification.

An older technique, used for more than 50 years, is photosuperimposition, in which a photograph of the possible individual is overlaid with a photographic transparency of the skull, which has been scaled to size and orientated to match the angle of the head in the portrait. If they do not fit, the lack of correspondence is usually obvious and any exclusion obtained can be as valuable as a positive identification. If the two images do fit together, by correspondence of anatomical landmarks such as chin, nasion, teeth, supraorbital ridges, external meatus etc., it is possible to say that the two images could have come from the same person, although identity cannot be fully established by the use of this method alone. Recently, this procedure has been refined by merging the two images on a television screen, which has the advantage that the images, particularly the portrait, can be manipulated prior to attempts at superimposition.

Chapter eight

Blood Stains

The distribution and appearance of the blood stains at the scene are now usually the province of specially trained and experienced forensic scientists, who will examine the scene specifically for these stains. The subject of blood-stain patterns has moved outside the normal sphere of expertise of a forensic medical practitioner; however, a sound knowledge of the principles is still essential for any doctor involved in legal matters.

BLOOD-STAIN PATTERNS

There are a number of different adjectives that can be used to describe how blood may flow from an injury – spurt, dribble, ooze etc. – and although it is obvious, medically, that damage to different types and sizes of blood vessels will result in different degrees of bleeding, it is extremely difficult to predict the exact type of flow of blood from an injury. In general terms, damage to an uncovered superficial artery is very likely to result in blood spurting some distance from the wound, whereas damage to a similarly sited vein will result in blood merely welling up out of the wound without any projectile force.

It is also important to remember that there is commonly a slight delay between the infliction of an injury that breaks the skin surface and blood appearing in the wound, as the vessels usually go into spasm for a second or two after the injury. The site of blood staining may therefore not necessarily be the site of infliction of the injury. Other complications include the presence

or absence of clothing and concurrent movement of the body or limb.

Blood spattering or splashing at a scene may have causes other than the simple flow from a wound, and distribution is also commonly either due to blood being thrown off by some active movement of the victim or a weapon or the result of simple dripping under the influence of gravity.

Active movement of the victim may result in dispersal of blood and this is most likely to occur when it is the limbs that are blood stained, as they can be moved faster. If the hand of a victim or assailant comes into contact with any bleeding wound, spots of blood can be thrown off the fingers when the arm is moved vigorously. Other blood stains may be caused by a victim coughing blood, which may have passed into the mouth from a bleeding nose or from a chest wound or even from a haematemesis.

Blood may also be dispersed by movement of a blood-stained weapon, whether sharp or blunt. It is, however, unlikely that the first injury will result in sufficient contamination of the weapon and it is the second and subsequent injuries that are associated with this type of blood dispersal. Different patterns of dispersal are found when blows are struck onto already blood-stained areas of the body; once again, it is the second and subsequent blows that are important.

The pattern a drop of blood makes when it strikes a surface depends on the angle of impact. If it hits at right angles, a circular stain is formed, spiked edges giving the spot a 'crown' appearance that suggests the contact was forcible. If the blood drop strikes obliquely, a tapering or 'tear-drop' stain is formed, the sharp end

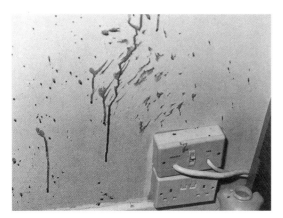

Figure 8.1 Pattern of blood splashes coughed by a man who had been stabbed in the chest. Note that many drops have struck the wall tangentially and that the larger drops have dribbled downwards.

pointing away from the origin and in the direction of travel. Sometimes there is also a small separate spot present in front of the sharp end of the stain, causing a shape to appear like an 'exclamation mark'.

Many blood stains are not due to blood drops flying freely through the air but are from direct contact with blood-stained areas of the body. Smearing indicates movement of the blood-stained object across the surface. Occasionally, a pattern may be left which may help to indicate the shape of a weapon, and fingerprints in blood are of particular importance.

When dribbles of blood are seen on the skin or clothing, common sense will indicate the posture of the individual. For example, a person bleeding while lying on his back will show trails of blood passing vertically backwards, whereas if the victim had remained erect, the blood will run downwards along the axis of the body.

Recent blood stains are usually obvious and very recent stains will show the striking red of oxygenated haemoglobin, but the age of a blood stain is difficult to assess with any degree of accuracy and a stain will rapidly lose this initial bright-red colour within hours and become a dull red; within days it will become brownish.

TESTS FOR BLOOD

As blood stains dry and age, their origin becomes less obvious and old blood stains may be mimicked by many other pigments. Sampling the stain must be done with care because not only its origin but also its site and appearance may be of importance. The position of the stain must first be marked and photographed and then the stain should either be scraped or rubbed off hard surfaces using a clean filter paper or soaked off absorbent surfaces using distilled water or saline.

The most sensitive tests are those for peroxidase activity of the haemoglobin molecule, using orthotolidine, phenolphthalein or benzidene (now banned in many countries because of its carcinogenic properties) and hydrogen peroxide. The current technique is the (Kastle–Meyer (KM) test, which will detect one part of blood in several millions. The mixed KM reagent (see Appendix 2) is added either to the material that has either been scraped onto a clean filter paper or to the stain extract, and an almost instant strong pink colour indicates the probability of blood being present. If the reagent has been prepared using benzidene and acetic acid, an instant, intense deep-blue colour indicates that the sample may contain blood. With either test, absence of a colour change indicates the absence of blood, but a positive reaction, though strongly suggestive that the material is blood, is not conclusive proof.

More specific methods include the Takayama test for producing haemochromogen crystal from haemoglobin and spectroscopic tests for haematin or methaemoglobin, and other chemical techniques can be applied in the laboratory.

SPECIES SPECIFICITY

A common alibi given by a suspect whose clothes or possessions have been blood stained is that he had been cutting meat or skinning rabbits etc. The KM test and the other tests noted above cannot distinguish human from animal blood and, apart from the rare exception of identifying the oval erythrocytes of the camel or the nucleated erythrocytes of birds and reptiles, there is nothing that can be done at the scene to confirm that the blood is human. This test requires laboratory facilities for immunological tests using specific antisera for various animals that have been raised in rabbits.

Chapter nine

The Examination of Wounds

Any doctor may be called upon to examine an individual who has sustained a wound as a result of an accident, an act of self-harm or from an action by a third party. It is essential that the doctor examines all wounds carefully and describes them completely and correctly. The examination and description of wounds can have far-reaching medico-legal implications, which may be civil or criminal and may not become apparent for many months or even years.

LAW ON WOUNDING

A 'wound' and an 'injury' are not distinguished in law, except in a charge of wounding where the skin must be 'breached'; such a definition would exclude rupture of the liver by a kick if the skin was not 'breached'.

An 'assault' is simply the threat of an attack and requires no physical contact; an actual attack involving contact is a 'battery'. In general parlance, however, the word 'assault' is commonly used to describe incidents with and without physical contact. Neither an assault nor a battery will necessarily result in a wound.

The term homicide encompasses not only murder but also several other types of non-accidental killing. The following broad categories are commonly found in legal codes, but the exact definitions and terminology will vary from jurisdiction to jurisdiction.

- *Murder*: this offence occurs when death follows the actions of an assailant who either intends to kill or intends to cause severe injury or is not concerned whether or not his actions will cause death or severe injury.
- *Manslaughter*: this is a lesser offence than murder and generally occurs when there is no intent to cause death or severe injury but where the death resulted from an unlawful act or gross negligence. Manslaughter may also be used when the assailant has been provoked by the victim or when the assailant suffers from a psychiatric disease such that he is incapable of forming the intent to kill. In some countries, causing death by the reckless driving of a motor vehicle is now a separate offence, distinguished from manslaughter.
- *Justifiable homicide*: this term applies to judicial executions in those countries where capital punishment is still allowed by law, and it can also be applied when an individual kills an assailant in order to defend himself or others when their lives are directly under a real, direct and immediate threat. In some countries, a police officer may also use lethal force to prevent the commission of a serious offence.

- *Infanticide*: this is the killing of an infant who is less than 1 year of age by the mother. Death may be due to an act of omission or commission when the balance of the mother's mind is disturbed by the effects of childbirth or lactation.

REPORTS

In these increasingly litigious times, it is important that doctors complete all medical notes with care, especially those that are likely to be examined in a court of law. In addition to recording the date, time and place of the examination, the doctor should also record, without comment, the history as related by the patient. A full examination of the patient should then be performed unless it is clear that injury is located in a few areas only. A contemporaneous note of the type, size, shape and position of the injuries with reference to fixed anatomical landmarks should be made.

TERMINOLOGY

The words used to describe injuries are important. The specialized medical meaning of words must only be used correctly and not in the 'lay' sense; for instance, the term 'laceration' must only be used to describe a break in the continuity of the skin caused by blunt trauma. If in doubt, it is better to use the lay words of cut, bruise, graze etc. when describing the nature of the wounds than to use medical terminology incorrectly. The courts consider it reasonable to expect that if doctors use specific medical terminology when writing a professional report, they will understand the terms they have used and they will have used those terms correctly.

The phase of recording information is a simple factual step; it does not require any specialist knowledge and it should be within the competence of any qualified medical practitioner. It may be that a doctor with no specialist forensic training will feel insufficiently qualified to interpret the wounds and, if so, he should resist any request to do so and should suggest that someone with greater experience in this field should provide that opinion. If he does not accept his limitations at this early stage, they may be demonstrated to him during cross-examination.

WOUNDS

Types of wound

Wounds caused by the application of physical force can be divided into two main groups: blunt force trauma and sharp force trauma. A third group of wounds is caused by the application of other forces that do not require movement or motion to produce their effects (Table 9.1).

Blunt force trauma is caused when an object, usually without a sharp or cutting edge, impacts the body or the body impacts the object. Three types of injury may result from such an impact: abrasions, contusions and lacerations.

Sharp force trauma occurs when an object with a sharp or sharpened edge impacts the body. The type of injury caused in this case depends upon the depth of the wound: an incised wound is longer than it is deep, whereas a stab wound is deeper than it is long.

Non-motion trauma is the third type of wounding. This type of wounding occurs when tissues, usually the epidermis or the mucosal surfaces, are damaged by direct application of a non-physical force, which can be thermal, chemical, electrical or electromagnetic.

Blunt force wounds

ABRASIONS

An abrasion is the most superficial type of injury and affects only the epidermis. As the epidermis does not contain blood vessels, abrasions should not bleed, but the folded nature of the junction between the dermis and the epidermis and the presence of loops of blood vessels in the dermal folds will mean that deep abrasions have a typical punctate or spotty appearance.

Table 9.1 Classification of Injuries

Kinetic injuries	Non-kinetic injuries
Blunt force injuries	Thermal: heat or cold
Abrasions	Chemical
Contusions	Electrical: high or low voltage
Lacerations	Electromagnetic
Sharp force injuries	
Incised wounds	
Stab wounds	

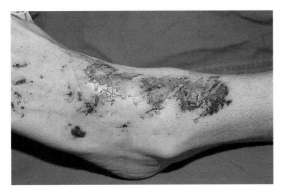

Figure 9.1 Abrasions from scraping against a rough surface during a fall.

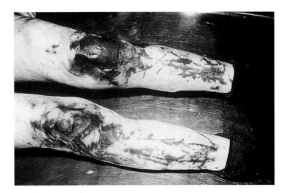

Figure 9.2 Extensive abrasions caused by stumbling, drunk and naked, against furniture. The dark leathery appearance is due to post-mortem drying of the damaged areas of skin.

Abrasions are usually caused by tangential glancing impacts but they can also be caused by crushing of the skin when the force is applied vertically down onto the skin. Bite marks and the grooved and often parchmented abrasion found in hanging are typical of crush abrasions.

The size, shape and type of abrasion depend upon the nature of the surface of the object which contacts the skin, its shape and the angle at which contact is made. Contact with the squared corner of an object (e.g. a brick) may well result in a linear abrasion, whereas contact with a side of the same object will cause a larger area of abrasion.

Contact with a large rough surface, such as a road, especially when associated with the higher levels of force found in traffic accidents, will result in much broader areas of abrasion, sometimes called 'brush abrasions' or 'gravel rash'.

Tangential contact with a smooth surface may well result in such fine, closely associated linear abrasions that the skin may simply appear reddened and roughened. This may be termed a 'friction burn'; close inspection will reveal the true nature of the wound.

The direction of the causative force can be identified by inspecting the wound – with a hand lens if necessary – and identifying the torn fragments of the epidermis which are pushed towards the furthest (distal) end of the abrasion.

Crush abrasions are important because they retain the pattern of the causative object. Diagrams and sketches can be extremely useful and, if possible, scaled photographs should be taken. Many different objects have been identified in this way: car radiator grills, the tread of escalator steps, plaited whips and the lines from floor tiles.

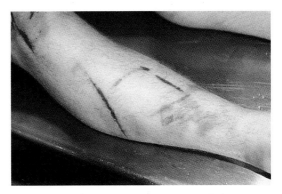

Figure 9.3 Mixed patterned abrasions due to impact with a vehicle bumper.

CONTUSIONS

Two events must occur before a contusion can form: the rupture of a blood vessel and the leakage of blood from the site of rupture into the surrounding tissues. Bruising is most commonly seen in the skin, but it can also occur in the deeper tissues, including muscle and internal organs.

The blood vessels that rupture are usually the small arteries and veins. Bleeding from ruptured capillaries would be so insignificant that it can be discounted in the formation of a bruise. The extent of the damage to the blood vessels is proportionate to the force applied: in general terms, the greater the force, the more blood vessels are damaged, the greater the leakage of blood and the bigger the bruise.

The blood leaks into the tissues along the fascial planes and so a bruise will not reliably reproduce the object which caused it and, as a bruise ages, the spread of the blood and so the relationship between the size and shape of the bruise and the causative object reduce.

There is one exception, which is the very superficial bruise caused by a moderate force where the leakage of blood is confined to the epidermis and the upper strata of the dermis, sometimes referred to as 'intradermal' bruises. In these bruises, the leakage of blood is small and the blood is held where it has leaked. As a result, these intradermal bruises can reproduce the nature of the object that caused them. Intradermal bruises are often associated with diffuse compression forces such as pressure from a car tyre or from a shoe during a stamp or a kick.

Bruises are not static. Their major component, blood, is both fluid and biodegradable and, as a result, bruises will change with time and under the influence of gravity. Indeed, some deep bruises (especially those to the deep muscles of the thigh) may 'come out' at the knee.

Once outside the confines of the blood vessel, blood is considered by the tissues to be foreign and they immediately begin to degrade and remove it. This degradation results in the colour change of a bruise that is so well known. In general terms, a bruise will initially be blue/dark blue/purple (depending on the amount of blood within the tissues) and it will then change to brown to green to yellow as the haemoglobin passes through various stages of degradation. Eventually, all of the blood is removed and the skin returns to its normal colour.

The speed of these changes is variable and it is not possible to use the colour changes as a 'clock' or 'timetable' of the bruise. Even in one individual, two bruises inflicted at the same time may differ in their appearances during resolution. The size of the bruise, the age of the individual (in older people bruises resolve more slowly), the presence of disease and many drugs may affect both the formation and the resolution of a bruise.

As a very broad rule of thumb, a small bruises in a fit young adult will resolve in about 1 week. Research in the 1980s showed that if yellow was identified, the bruise was over 18 hours old, whereas if no yellow could be seen, the bruise could not be reliably aged. It is to be hoped that further research will elucidate this matter.

It is essential to remember that the skin from Asians, Africans and blacks has a layer of melanin pigment of varying intensity. This will reduce the visibility of a bruise and will mask the colour changes that occur. In the examination of a living victim with dark skin, a bruise may only be identified by palpation. Pathologically, it is possible to identify bruising by dissection and inspection of the undersurface of the skin.

Bruising can occur after death: the blood vessels are just as easily damaged by the application of force and, providing there is blood with some pressure within those vessels, bruising can occur. Such pressure may exist at the lowermost vessels due to the static weight of the column of blood. Post-mortem bruises are generally small and lie on the dependent parts of the body. Bruising may also be found in the areas of post-mortem dissection and care must be taken in interpreting new bruises when an autopsy has been performed.

Although bruises do not reflect with any accuracy the object causing them, there are some particular patterns that indicate the type of weapon used. One such pattern is the 'tramline' or 'railway line' bruise caused by a blow from a linear object. This pattern occurs because the major stretching and shearing of the skin occur at the edges of contact and not directly beneath the centre of the object, which is simply compressed. Impact by a hard ball produces concentric rings of bruising for similar reasons.

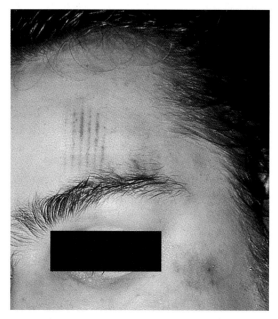

Figure 9.4 Patterned intradermal bruise on the forehead due to a fall onto ribbed ceramic tiles.

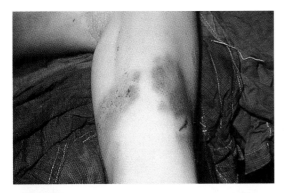

Figure 9.5 Bruising of the upper arm. The pattern of these bruises is typical of forceful gripping. Small abrasions from fingernails are also seen.

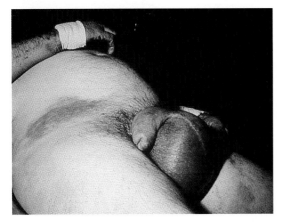

Figure 9.6 Recent bruising of the abdominal wall and scrotum due to kicking.

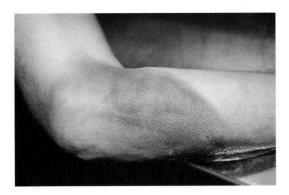

Figure 9.7 Colour changes in a bruise. This injury is reported to be 10 days old and contains brown, blue and purple components.

The patterns of bruises are extremely important: a row of oval or round bruises may be due to impact by the knuckles in a punch; groups of small oval or round bruises are also indicative of fingertip pressure as in

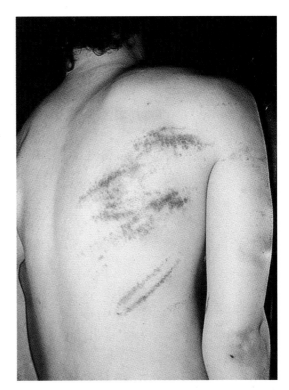

Figure 9.8 Typical 'railway-line' bruises caused by a wooden rod. Note that the centre of the parallel contusions is unmarked.

gripping and there is sometimes a single, larger, thumb bruise on the opposite side of the limb. Fingertip bruises on the neck or along the jaw line are commonly seen in manual strangulation.

LACERATIONS

Lacerations are the result of a blunt force overstretching the skin and the result is a split, which usually passes through the full thickness of the skin. A laceration is deep and will bleed. Because the skin is composed of many different tissues, some of the more resilient tissues will not be damaged by the forces that split the weaker tissues. These most resilient tissues are often nerves, the small fibrous bands of the fascial planes and, sometimes, at the base of the laceration, the occasional medium-sized elastic blood vessels. These fibres arch across the defect in the skin and are referred to as 'bridging fibres'.

Lacerations are most common where the skin can be compressed between the applied force and underlying bone (i.e. over the scalp, face, elbows, knees, shins etc). They are rare (unless severe force has been applied)

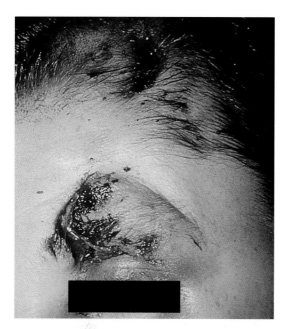

Figure 9.9 Laceration of eyebrow due to impact on the edge of a brick. The wound has clean edges but the abraded margins can be seen.

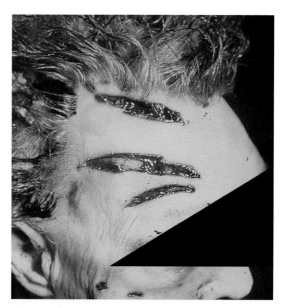

Figure 9.11 Multiple lacerations from a blunt steel bar. These were initially mistaken by the police for axe wounds. The abraded or crushed margins can be easily seen.

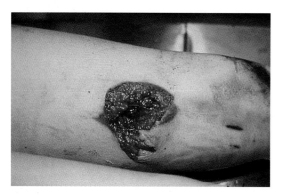

Figure 9.10 Laceration of an arm of a pedestrian struck by a car. The impact has been oblique, causing a flap of skin to tear away to the right.

over the soft, fleshy areas of the body such as the buttocks, breasts and abdomen.

When the force applied to the skin is more tangential, as in the rolling or grinding action of a vehicle wheel, the laceration may be horizontal and result in a large area of separation of skin from the underlying tissues. This can be termed 'flaying'.

The margins of a laceration are always ragged; however, if a thin regular object inflicts an injury over a bony area of the body, the wound caused may look very sharply defined and can be mistaken for an incised injury. Careful inspection of the margins will reveal some crushing and bruising, and examination of the inner surfaces of the wound will reveal the presence of bridging fibres.

The laceration may reflect the object causing it if that object is straight, but this wound is a poor reproducer in other circumstances.

Sharp force wounds

INCISED WOUNDS

Incised wounds are caused by objects with a sharp or cutting edge, most commonly a knife but an axe, shards of glass, broken glasses and bottles, an edge of broken pottery, a piece of metal etc. can also cause these wounds. An incised injury is distinguished from a stab wound by being longer than it is deep.

The edges of the wound will give some indication as to the sharpness of the weapon causing it. A sharp edge will leave no bruising or abrasion of the wound margins. Careful inspection of the internal structure of the wound will reveal that no bridging fibres are present because the cutting edge divides everything in its passage into the skin.

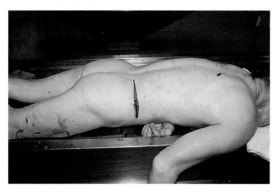

Figure 9.12 Incised wound to the flank; it is clearly longer than it is deep.

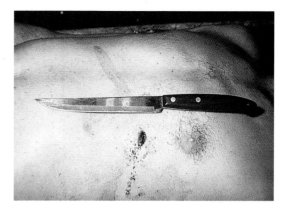

Figure 9.13 Fatal stab wound of the chest and the knife that caused it. The wound does not reproduce the size of the knife, due to contraction of the elastic fibres in the skin.

Incised wounds, by their nature, are rarely life threatening because they seldom penetrate deeply enough to damage a blood vessel of significant size. However, incised wounds over the wrist or neck, where major arteries lie in the superficial tissues, can prove fatal.

STAB WOUNDS

A stab wound is deeper than it is long and it is the depth of the injury that makes it so often fatal and hence of such forensic interest. Stabbing is the commonest method of homicide in Britain and accounts for over 50 per cent of all murders, many of which are domestic in type.

Any weapon with a point or tip can cause a stab wound; the edge of the blade does not need to be sharp. For penetration to occur, the tip must be pressed against the skin with sufficient force to overcome the natural elasticity of the skin. The factors that determine how much force is needed for penetration to occur are:

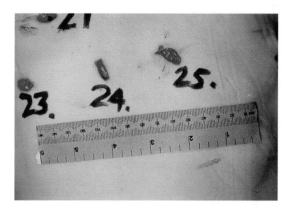

Figure 9.14 Multiple stab wounds from the same weapon as in Fig. 9.13, showing marked variation in size and appearance.

- The sharpness of the tip of the weapon: the sharper the tip, the easier it is to penetrate the skin.
- The speed of the contact: the faster the contact, the greater the force applied and the easier it is to penetrate the skin.
- Whether clothing has been penetrated: clothing increases the resistance to penetration.
- Whether bone or cartilage has been injured: skin offers very little resistance to a stabbing action by a sharp knife, but penetration of these denser tissues will require greater force.

Experiments have shown that once a knife has penetrated the skin, the rest of the weapon follows with

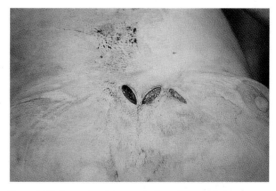

Figure 9.15 A complex stab wound where all three injuries are caused by a single action. The first entry is in the right breast; there is an exit wound in the middle and a re-entry wound over the centre of the chest.

almost no additional force being applied. In his text-book *Forensic Pathology*, Knight says that he believes this is because the skin indents before penetration and acts as a reservoir of energy. The insertion of a sharp knife into the body, especially through the skin stretched across ribs, requires very little force, and pressure from a single finger is sufficient to push a sharp scalpel through the chest wall at this site. With these factors in mind, it is clear that it is possible, in some circumstances, for a person to transfix himself by walking or falling onto the tip of a sharp weapon. No forward movement of the weapon is necessary and, according to Knight, the hand or arm holding the knife does not need to be braced or fixed for penetration to occur.

The commonest weapon used is a knife of some sort, but swords, shards of glass, broken bottles etc. can be used and even screwdrivers, metal rods, railings etc. can all cause stab wounds if sufficient force is applied.

The appearances of a stab wound on the skin will reflect, but not necessarily mimic, the cross-sectional shape of the weapon used. If a blade of some sort is used, the following general comments apply.

- A slit-like wound will distort after removal of the weapon by the action of the elastic fibres present in the skin. If the fibres run at right angles to the wound, it will be pulled outwards and get shorter and wider; if they run parallel to the wound, it will be pulled lengthways and the edges will tend to close and the wound elongate slightly.
- Even if the edges of the wound are gently pushed together, the resulting defect is seldom the same size as the knife, and personal experience suggests that the wounds and the weapon may differ by up to ± 1 cm.
- The size of the wound also depends on the shape of the blade and how deeply it was inserted.
- Movement of the knife in the wound, either by the assailant 'rocking' it or by the victim moving to escape, will cause the wound to be enlarged. If the knife is twisted or rotated, a triangular wound may be caused.
- Many knives have only one cutting edge, the other being blunt. This design may be reproduced in the wound where one 'V'-shaped sharp point can be seen and one blunt point. The blunt point may split and a tiny spike or triangle is sometimes formed, which is often referred to as a 'fishtail'.
- If the knife is fully inserted, bruising or abrasion of the skin adjacent to the stab wound caused by a hilt

of the weapon or by the hand of the assailant can be seen provided that clothing has not intervened.

- The depth of a wound can be greater than the length of the blade if a forceful stab is inflicted. This is because the abdomen and, to a lesser extent, the chest can be compressed by the force of the hilt or hand against the skin.
- A blunt object such as a screwdriver or spike will tend to indent, split and bruise the skin on insertion. Different types of screwdriver will cause different patterns of injury. Cross-head or 'Phillips' screwdrivers cause very distinctive cruciate skin wounds.
- Sharp but irregular instruments such as scissors or chisels will leave particular patterns of injury, with a 'Z' shape from scissors and a rectangular shape from a chisel. If the stab wounds are unusual, it is important to consider unusual instruments.

PATTERNS OF INJURY

The three possible motives for infliction of a wound apply and there can be little to distinguish between accidental and deliberate infliction by simply examination of a single wound. However, examination of the site, orientation and pattern(s) of the wounds will often reveal useful indications about the causation of the wound.

Particular actions result in particular and often identifiable patterns of injury. Punches, kick, bites, holding or gripping injuries and defence injuries can be identified by their patterns.

A punch is a blow delivered by the clenched fist. The blow can be directed anywhere, but usually leaves a wound only over those areas of the body where the skin is closely applied to bone, as in the face and skull. The wounds caused are bruises, abrasions and, where the skin is over an edge such as the eyebrow or cheeks, lacerations. The lips can also be forced back onto the teeth, resulting in lacerations inside the lips.

Bones may be broken, but punches will usually affect only the thinner bones such as the nose or vulnerable flat bones such as the mandible and the maxilla. Ribs may be fractured by blows of sufficient force.

Contusions of the face may result in extensive spreading of the blood, and periorbital haematomas (black eyes) are common, although it is important to remember that fractures of the nose can also result in haematomas at these sites.

In the very young and old, intra-abdominal injury, including mesenteric laceration, intestinal rupture and injury to the major abdominal organs, may rarely occur.

Kicking and stamping injuries are caused by a foot which is either swung or moved downwards with some force. These actions can deliver blunt force trauma to the body and, as a result, abrasions, contusions and lacerations may result. There are some minor differences between the modes of application of force and, as stamping injuries have a more compressive component, they may result in more bruises and lacerations with fewer abrasions. Stamping injuries, particularly those caused by 'trainers', may leave areas of intra-dermal bruising that reflect the pattern of the sole of the shoe.

The victim is often on the ground when these injuries are inflicted, and blows from the foot are commonly directed towards the head and face, the chest and the abdomen. The high levels of force that can be applied by a foot mean that there are often underlying skeletal injuries. These are most common in the facial skeleton and in the ribs. Stamping injuries to the front of the abdomen may result in rupture of the internal organs, particularly the liver and the spleen.

Bite marks are crush abrasions. They are commonly associated with bruising and may be associated with lacerations if severe force is applied. Bite marks can be seen in sexual assaults, child abuse and occasionally on the sports field.

Bite marks are commonly composed of a pair of curved lines of bruises facing towards each other. Inspection may reveal distinctive linear crush abrasions indicating the patterns of the teeth. Attempts at identification of the assailant should be left to an odontologist.

Bite marks may be found on almost any surface of the body; specific sites are associated with specific forms of assault. The neck, breasts and shoulders are often bitten in a sexually motivated attack, while in child abuse bites of the arms and the buttocks are common. Adolescent self-inflicted bites can be seen on the medial aspect of the arm.

Bites can also be inflicted by many common inhabitants of a house, including family pets. Odontological examination will reveal different sizes, different arch shapes and different dentition in these cases.

If a suspected bite is found at examination, a swab of the area should be taken for DNA and the bite should be photographed with a scale. Photography using ultraviolet light may be of assistance in older cases.

Defence injuries are caused as victims try to defend themselves against an attack. The type of injury caused depends upon the weapon used and the force applied: an attack by a blunt weapon may result in bruises on

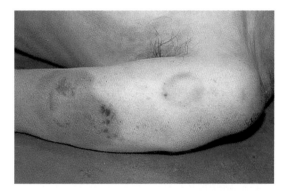

Figure 9.17 Bite marks on the arm. The upper bite shows abrasion and bruising from the opposing dental arches. In the diffuse bruising of the lower arm, a group of abrasions caused by the incisors can be seen.

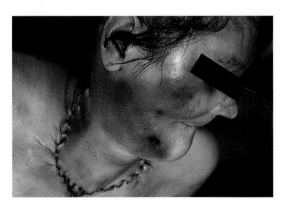

Figure 9.16 Extensive bruising and abrasion of the face due to kicking.

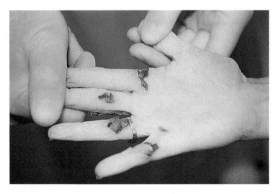

Figure 9.18 Defence wounds on the palmar surface of the hand caused by attempts to grasp or deflect a blade.

LIVERPOOL JOHN MOORES UNIVERSITY
LEARNING SERVICES

the ulnar (little finger) side of the forearm where it was raised to protect the head and face. Defence against a sharp weapon may result in incised and stab wounds to the ulnar aspect of the forearm or across the palm of the hand and the palmar aspect of the fingers.

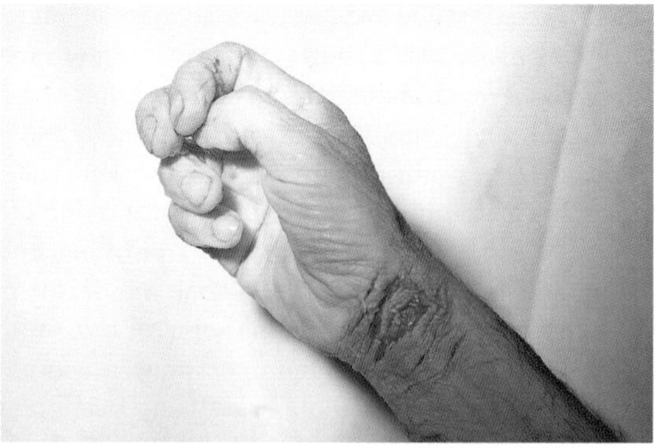

SURVIVAL

The length of survival following receipt of an injury is always difficult to determine: every human being is different and this variability in survival and post-injury activity is to be expected. Any expression of either survival time or of the ability to move and react must be given on the basis of the 'most likely' scenario, accepting that many different versions are possible. The court should be advised of the difficulties of this assessment and should be encouraged also to consider the eyewitness accounts.

It must be remembered that survival for a time after injury and long-term survival are not one and the same thing. The initial response of the body to haemorrhage is compensatable shock, but if blood loss continues, the homeostatic mechanisms may be overwhelmed and the individual enters the phase of non-compensatable shock, which leads inexorably to death.

SELF-INFLICTED INJURIES

All types of injury can be self-inflicted, accidentally inflicted or deliberately inflicted by another.

In broad terms, self-inflicted blunt injuries are caused by jumping from a height or under a train etc. and there are no specific features of the injuries that identify them as self-inflicted. Self-inflicted bite marks may occasionally be seen on the arms of an individual who claims to have been assaulted.

Self-inflicted incised or stabbing injuries, on the other hand, do show specific patterns and the patterns vary depending on the aim of the individual. In sui-cidal individuals, self-inflicted sharp force injuries are most commonly found at specific sites on the body called the 'elective sites' – for incised wounds these are most commonly on the front of the wrists and neck, whereas stabbing injuries are most commonly found over the precordium and the abdomen. In individuals who only desire to 'self-harm' or mutilate themselves,

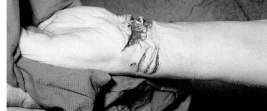

Figure 9.19 Self-inflicted incised wounds have the typical appearance of multiple, superficial and parallel incised injuries.

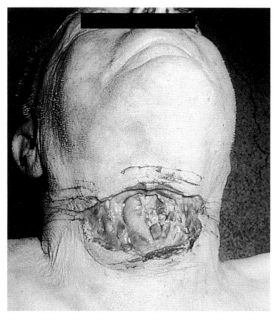

Figure 9.20 Multiple tentative or hesitation injuries of the wrist typical of self-infliction.

Figure 9.21 Tentative injuries in self-inflicted injury to the elective site on the neck.

the site can be anywhere on the body that can be reached by the individual. Except in cases of severe mental disease, the eyes, lips, nipples and genitalia tend to be spared.

The other features of self-inflicted injuries lie in the multiple, predominantly parallel nature of the wounds and, in suicidal acts, the more superficial injuries are referred to as 'hesitation' or 'tentative' injuries.

LIVERPOOL
JOHN MOORES UNIVERSITY
AVRIL ROBARTS LRC
TITHEBARN STREET
LIVERPOOL L2 2ER
TEL. 0151 231 4022

Regional Injuries

Many injuries, or rather their effects, will vary depending on the exact area of the body that is injured. A stab wound to a limb is unlikely to have fatal consequences, whereas a similar injury to the chest may well be fatal. Similarly, the effects of a blow to the chest may be minimal but the consequences of exactly the same blow to the head may be catastrophic.

HEAD INJURIES

Injuries to the head are particularly important because of the brain's vital role in sustaining the life of the individual. The brain is protected within the strong, bony skull, but it is not well restrained within this compartment and injuries to the brain result from differences between the motion of the skull and the brain. There are three main components of the head: the scalp, the skull and the brain.

Scalp

The scalp is vascular, hair-bearing skin; at its base is a thick fibrous membrane called the galea aponeurotica. Lying between the galea and the skull is a very thin sheet of connective tissue that is penetrated by blood vessels (emissary veins) emerging through the skull, and beneath this connective tissue is the periosteum of the outer table of the skull.

The vascularity of the scalp, possibly the connection with the intracranial blood vessels, results in profuse bleeding if it is injured. Bleeding will also, very commonly, continue after death if the head is in a dependent position.

The scalp is easily injured by blunt trauma as it can be crushed between the weapon and the underlying skull, which acts like an anvil. Bruises of the scalp are associated with prominent oedema because this normal tissue response cannot spread and dissipate as easily as in other areas of the body. The easiest way to detect scalp injuries is by palpation, but shaving is essential for proper documentation and photography.

Lacerations of the scalp will, if inspected carefully, reveal a band of abrasion adjacent to the laceration, and examination of the depths of the wound will reveal the bridging fibres that will confirm the true origin of these injuries. This is important because the relative thinness of the scalp and its immobility mean that blunt trauma can result in sharply defined injuries that may, at first sight, appear to be incised injuries.

Tangential forces or glancing blows, either from an instrument or from a rotating wheel as in a road traffic accident, may tear large flaps of tissue, exposing the underlying skull. If hair becomes entangled in rotating machinery, portions of the scalp may be avulsed.

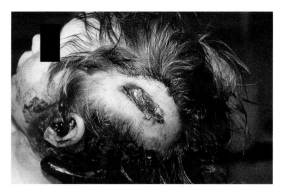

Figure 10.1 A laceration of the scalp caused by a linear, blunt object – a metal bar. The abrasion of the edges of the wound can be clearly seen.

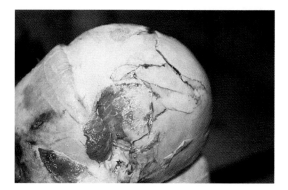

Figure 10.3 Interlacing fractures of the skull from repeated blows to the head (as Fig. 10.2).

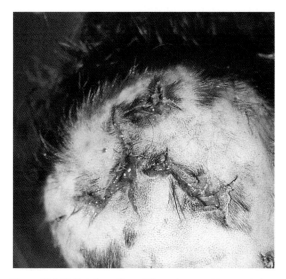

Figure 10.2 Multiple lacerations of the scalp caused by repeated blows from a blunt object. Abrasion of the margins is not as pronounced as in Fig. 10.1.

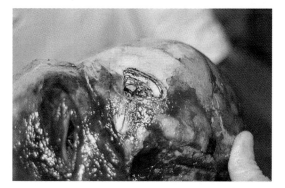

Figure 10.4 Depressed fracture of the skull caused by an oblique hammer blow. Note the fan-shaped defect with terraced splintering. The head was in a black plastic bag when struck and portions of this material can be seen in the fissures.

Skull fractures

The skeleton of the human head is complex and can be divided into three components: the mandible, the facial skeleton and the closed container that contains the brain – the calvaria. The calvaria is composed of eight plates of bone, each of varying thickness, with buttresses passing through and across the bony margins. The skull is designed in part to protect the brain and in part to provide a mobile but secure platform for the receptor organs of the special senses.

The mechanism of formation of skull fractures is extremely complex. It has been extensively studied and much is now known about the way the skull behaves when forces are applied. Simply put, the skull is not an entirely rigid structure and it is able to bend and distort when force is applied to it. If the forces applied exceed the ability of the skull to distort, fractures will occur. However, fractures will represent the point of maximum stress upon the skull, which may not be at the immediate site of impact. The skulls of infants and children are thinner than those of adults and may be able to distort more before breaking.

Apart from depressed fractures underlying major, localized areas of trauma, skull fractures are seldom, of themselves, life threatening. The crucial feature of skull fractures is that they are a marker for the application of severe force to the head. It is the effects upon the brain that are important, and severe brain injury can occur in the absence of any bony injury. Unfortunately for the practice of forensic medicine, the converse may also be true and skull fractures can be caused with no obvious evidence of injury to the brain or neurological defect – however, the larger the fracture the less likely this is to be true.

A pathologist can only make broad comments about the possible effect upon an individual of a blow to the head. As with all injuries, a spectrum of effects is to be expected if a large number of people were to receive exactly the same injury in exactly the same way.

If localized force is applied to the skull, the fractures will form at the sites of maximum force and so can be a useful guide to the position and nature of the instrument. In general, however, the wound to the scalp will usually have identified point(s) of contact.

Blows to the top of the head commonly result in long linear fractures that pass down the parietal plates and may, if the force was severe, pass inwards across the floor of the skull, usually beside the sphenoid bone in the middle fossa. If the fractures extend from both sides, they may join at the pituitary fossa and produce a complete fracture across the floor of the skull – a hinge fracture. This type of fracture indicates the application of severe force and may be seen in traffic accidents or falls from high buildings.

Falls from a height onto the top of the skull or onto the feet, where the force is transmitted to the base of the brain through the spine, may result in ring fracture of the base of the skull around the foramen magnum, whereas localized blows to the large bony plates, particularly the parietal bones, may result in a 'spider's web' type of fracture composed of radiating lines transected by concentric circles.

Depressed fractures will force fragments of skull inwards and, due to the bilayer construction of the skull, the inner table fragmentation will be much greater than the fracturing of the outer table, and fragments of bone can be driven into the underlying meninges, blood vessels and brain tissue.

The orbital plates, the upper surfaces of the orbits within the skull, are composed of extremely thin sheets of bone which are easily fractured, and these 'blow-out' fractures may be the only indication of the application of significant force to the skull.

Special mention must be made of skull fractures in children and infants. These fractures are extremely important forensically but their interpretation can be extremely difficult. It is self-evident that skull fractures may be the result of either deliberate or accidental acts and differentiation must depend on the consideration of as much relevant information as possible (see Chapter 20).

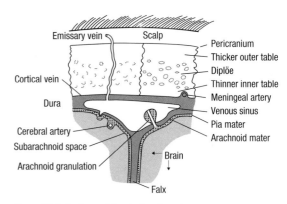

Figure 10.5 Anatomy of the skull and meninges.

Intracranial haemorrhage

Haemorrhages within the cranial cavity have a particular significance in forensic medicine and they are the cause of many deaths and disability following head injury. Bleeding into the closed cranial cavity results in the development of a space-occupying mass, which will compress and move the brain and which will, if bleeding continues for sufficient time and if sufficient blood accumulates, raise the pressure within the cranial cavity. As the intracranial pressure increases, the blood flow to the brain decreases. If the intracranial pressure reaches a point where it equals or exceeds arterial blood pressure, the blood flow to the brain will cease.

The anatomy of the blood vessels within the skull has a major influence on the type of bleeding that will occur with different types of trauma. The meningeal arteries run in grooves in the inner table of the skull and lie outside the dura. They are generally protected from the shearing effect of sudden movement but are damaged by fracture lines that cross their course. The venous sinuses lie within the dura and the connecting veins pass between the sinuses and the cortical veins; these vessels are not directly affected by skull fractures but are at risk when there is differential movement between the brain and the skull as in shearing. The true blood supply to the brain, the cerebral arteries and veins, lie beneath the arachnoid membrane and are protected from all but penetrating injuries.

There are two main causes of traumatic haemorrhage within the skull, each resulting in haemorrhage in different planes: extradural and subdural. Extradural haemorrhage is associated with damage to the meningeal artery, particularly the middle meningeal artery in its course in the temporal bone. Damage to

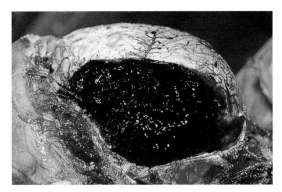

Figure 10.6 A large extradural haemorrhage caused by damage to the middle meningeal artery from a fracture of the temporal bone.

this vessel results in arterial bleeding into the extradural space. As the blood accumulates, it separates the dura from the overlying skull and forms a haematoma. Arterial bleeding is likely to be fast and the development of the haematoma will result in a rapid displacement of the brain and the rapid onset of symptoms. Rarely, extradural haemorrhage can develop as a result of venous bleeding from damaged perforating veins or dural sinuses, in which case the development of symptoms will be slower.

The second cause of traumatic intracranial haemorrhage is damage to the communicating veins as they cross the subdural space. This venous damage is not necessarily associated with fractures of the skull. In many instances, particularly in the very young and the very old, there may be no history or evidence of any trauma to the head. These venous injuries are associated with rotational or shearing forces that cause the brain to move relative to the inner surface of the skull; this motion stretches the thin-walled veins, causing them to rupture. The venous bleeding lies in the subdural space. Recent subdural haemorrhages are dark red in colour and shiny, but begin to turn brown after a few days; microscopically, haemosiderin can be identified with Perl's stain. Older subdural collections may be enclosed in gelatinous membranes, which can harden into a firm rubbery capsule in extreme cases. Such old collections of subdural blood are most commonly seen in the elderly, whose cerebral atrophy allows space for the formation of the haematoma without significant clinical effects. Occasionally, these subdurals may be many months or even years old. They may have been the cause of a change in neurological state that was variously ascribed to a stroke or the onset of a psychiatric condition.

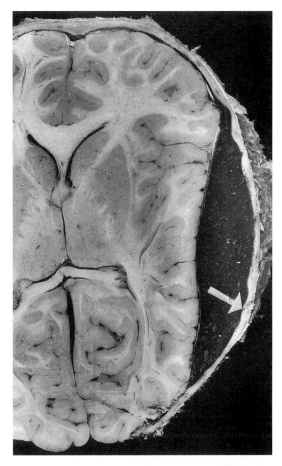

Figure 10.7 Fracture (arrowed) of the temporal bone resulting in tearing of the middle meningeal artery and a large extradural haemorrhage. Collapse occurred 4 hours after receiving a 'trivial' injury to the head.

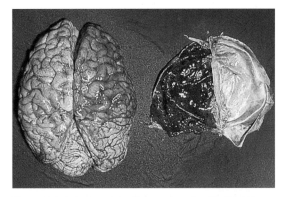

Figure 10.8 A chronic subdural haemorrhage found incidentally at autopsy of an elderly person who had died from other causes. The brown, gelatinous material is seen on the under-surface of the meninges.

EFFECTS

The effects of both extradural and subdural haemorrhages are essentially the same: they both act as space-occupying lesions compressing the brain and, at their most severe, causing herniation through the tentorium cerebelli. The speed at which symptoms develop is variable and both are associated with a period of apparent normality – the lucid period – after the injury and before the onset of neurological symptoms. In general terms, the arterial bleeding would be expected to produce symptoms and signs of raised intracranial pressure more quickly than the venous bleeding of the subdural haemorrhage.

Traumatic subarachnoid haemorrhage

Small areas of subarachnoid haemorrhage are common where there has been direct trauma to the brain, either from an intrusive injury such as a depressed fracture or from movement of the brain against the inner surface of the skull as a result of acceleration or deceleration injuries. These small injuries are usually associated with areas of underlying cortical contusion and sometimes laceration.

Large basal subarachnoid haemorrhages can be of traumatic origin and follow forceful blows or kicks to the neck, particularly to the upper neck adjacent to the ear, but any blow which results in rapid rotation or flexion of the neck can cause this damage. The vertebral arteries are confined within foraminae in the lateral margins of the upper six cervical vertebrae and are susceptible to trauma either with or without fracture of the foramina. It is thought that most of the damage to the arteries as a result of trauma occurs at the site at which they penetrate the spinal dura to enter the posterior fossa of the skull.

It must be remembered that basal subarachnoid haemorrhages are most commonly non-traumatic in origin and arise from the spontaneous rupture of a berry aneurysm of one of the arteries in the circle of Willis. Great care must be taken to exclude this natural cause.

Brain injury

Injuries that have resulted in skull fractures or intracranial haemorrhage are clear macroscopic markers that significant force has been applied to the head and therefore to the brain. Sometimes, however, these markers are absent but, as a result of acceleration or deceleration, the brain has been significantly traumatized. Whatever the exact cause of the trauma, the effects on the brain as a whole are the same and cerebral oedema develops. The mechanism of cerebral oedema is complex and not fully understood, but appears to be due to transudation of fluid into the extracellular space.

As oedema develops, the brain swells and, as the skull cannot expand to allow for the swelling, the intracranial pressure rises and the brain is squeezed out of the spaces in the meninges and the skull. The cerebrum is forced downwards through the tentorium cerebelli and the cerebellum and brainstem are forced downwards through the foramen magnum. These movements produce secondary areas of injury in the unci of the cerebrum and the cerebellar tonsils.

The weight of the oedematous brain is increased and the surface of the brain is markedly flattened, often with haemorrhage and necrosis of the unci and the cerebellar tonsils; sectioning reveals compression of the ventricles, sometimes into thin slits.

Direct injuries to the brain from depressed or comminuted skull fractures result in areas of bruising and laceration to the cortex, often associated with larger sites of haemorrhage. These injuries can occur at any site, above or below the tentorium. Penetrating injuries from gunshots or from stab wounds will cause injuries deep into the white matter, and the tissue adjacent to the wound tracks will often be associated with contusion.

There is also another group of injuries that are associated with head injuries, particularly the injuries that do not result in either penetration or intracranial haemorrhage. The brain is injured in these cases by rotation or by acceleration/deceleration, which causes shearing between the different layers or components of the brain as each moves in a different way or at a different speed. This shearing causes contusions and lacerations deep within the substance of the brain, but particularly in the region of the corpus callosum. Shearing is also associated with the so-called 'gliding lesions' that occur beneath the cortex and in the cerebral peduncles and brainstem.

The shearing effects are also identifiable at a microscopic level, where the damage to the axons can be identified by the use of special staining techniques. These changes have been termed diffuse axonal injury. They take a finite time to develop, or at least to become apparent, and in cases of immediate or very rapid death the microscopic changes may not be identifiable. Where there has been survival for an hour or so, βAPP (beta apoprotein precursor) may be identified in the axons of the damaged nerves by immunohistological techniques. At later stages, retraction balls may be identified by silver staining techniques.

COUP AND CONTRA COUP

The distinction between coup and contra-coup injuries to the brain has always been a point of considerable discussion, possibly because, if this separation of patterns of head injury can be made, then the forensic pathologist is able to form an opinion about the situation of the head at the time of the injury.

The key to this feature lies in the movement of the brain within the skull. A coup injury occurs when a static head is struck. This causes the skull to be accelerated and to strike the underlying brain and this results in direct trauma. The injury to the scalp will overlie the injury to the brain.

In contra coup, the skull and the brain are moving together and the skull is suddenly arrested. The major force will be one of deceleration and, in this situation, the injuries to the brain are found on the opposite side of the skull to the scalp injury. Typically, in a moving head striking the ground on the occipital region, the brain injuries are found on the tips of the temporal poles and in the subfrontal regions.

Because of the complex and variable shape of the skull, the pattern of contra-coup injuries is not always so easy to identify: a fall onto the frontal area is not associated with contra-coup injuries in the occipital region

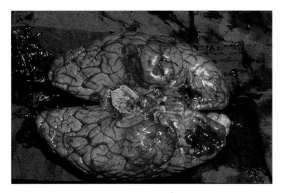

Figure 10.9 Classical contra-coup contusion of the subfrontal regions in a man who fell on to the back of his head.

and a fall onto the parietal regions may be associated with contusions in both the contralateral hemisphere and the medial aspect of the ipsilateral hemisphere adjacent to the falx.

NECK INJURIES

The neck can be, and often is, the site of many different types of injury. Its prominence in forensic medicine is due to two features: the presence of a large number of vital structures – throat and larynx, major blood vessels, major nerve trunks, the spine and the spinal cord – and the fact that it is of a size that can be grasped and easily held.

There are no specific features to mention regarding sharp force trauma or gunshot wounds to the neck. The application of pressure to the neck, whether by ligature or manually, results in a specialized group of injuries that are best considered with the other forms of asphyxiation in Chapter 13.

SPINAL INJURIES

The spine is a complex structure with interlocking but mobile components. It is designed to flex to a great extent but lateral movement and extension are much more limited. The spine is very commonly injured in major trauma such as road traffic accidents or falls from a height, and severe injury with discontinuity is easily identified. However, sometimes the spinal injuries are more subtle and it is only after careful dissection that damage to the upper cervical spine and, in particular, disruption of the atlanto-occipital joint will be revealed.

For the survivors of trauma, spinal injuries may have some of the most crucial long-term effects because the spinal cord is contained within the spinal canal and there is little, if any, room for movement of the canal before the cord is damaged. The sequelae of spinal damage will depend upon the exact site and the exact type of the injury.

The type of injury to the spine will depend upon the degree of force and the angle at which the spine is struck. A column is extremely strong in compression and, unless the force applied is so severe that the base of the skull is fractured, vertically applied forces will

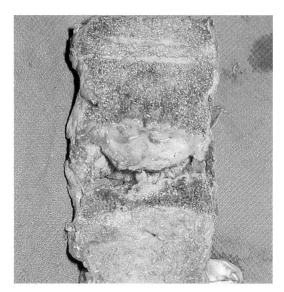

Figure 10.10 Crushed vertebral body due to a hyperflexion injury of the thoracic spine.

generally result in little damage if the spine is straight. Angulation of the spine will alter the transmission of force and will make the spine much more susceptible to injury, particularly at the site of the angulation.

Force applied to the spine may result in damage to the discs or to the vertebral bodies. The other major components of the vertebrae – the neural arches and the transverse processes – are more likely to be injured if the force of the trauma is not aligned with the spine.

Whiplash injuries associated with road traffic fatalities are very common and are due to the hyperextension of the neck, hyperflexion being less likely to cause damage. Hyperflexion injuries can be caused if heavy weights are dropped onto the back of a crouching individual; this scenario may be seen in roof falls in the mining industry.

Forceful extension of the spine can be seen, although rarely now, in the cervical injuries associated with judicial hanging where there is a long drop before the sudden arrest and forceful extension of the neck. Forceful flexion of the spine will commonly lead to the 'wedge' fracture or compression of the anterior aspect of a vertebral body. Lateral forces will lead to fracture dislocations where one vertebral body passes across its neighbour – this displacement will seriously compromise the vertebral canal. Damage to the intervertebral discs can occur as a solitary lesion or it may be part of a more complex spinal injury.

CHEST INJURIES

The chest can be subject to all kinds of injury and is particularly susceptible to both blunt and penetrating injuries.

Adequate respiration requires freedom of movement of the chest, functioning musculature and integrity of the chest wall. Any injury that impairs or prevents any of these activities will result in a reduction in the ability to breathe, which may result in asphyxiation. External pressure on the chest may result in traumatic asphyxia by restricting movement; this may occur during road traffic accidents or following collapse of structures such as mines etc. Pressure on the chest that restricts movement may also occur if the individual simply gets into, or is placed into, a position in which the free movement of the chest is restricted. This positional asphyxia occurs most commonly in individuals who are rendered immobile through alcohol or drugs, but may also be seen in those suffering from incapacitating neurological disease who are unable to extricate themselves from these positions (see Chapter 13).

Blunt injury may result in fractures of the ribs. The fracture of a few ribs is unlikely to have much effect, other than causing pain, in a fit adult. However, if there are numerous rib fractures, and particularly if they are adjacent, the structure of the chest wall may be compromised and it will not be able to function as the fixed structure required for respiration. Multiple rib fractures may result in the so-called 'flail' chest and, clinically, the area of chest around the fractures may be seen to move inwards on inspiration – paradoxical respiration. The clinical effects of such injuries depend on their extent and on the respiratory reserve of the individual: an elderly man with chronic lung disease may be tipped into terminal respiratory failure by injuries that would only be a painful irritant to a fit young man.

Rib fractures may have other more serious consequences. If the sharp ends of the fractured bones are driven inwards, they may penetrate the underlying lung, resulting in a pneumothorax. If subcostal or pulmonary blood vessels are also injured, the resulting haemorrhage associated with the leakage of air will produce a haemopneumothorax. Pneumothoraces may also develop if fractured rib margins are forced outwards through the skin.

Children are, in general, more resilient and better able to cope with rib fractures. However, rib fractures in children have a particular place in forensic medicine, as they are a marker for child abuse (see Chapter 20).

Rib fractures can also be artefactual and the use of cardiopulmonary resuscitation (CPR) or cardiac massage by both skilled and unskilled individuals has resulted in an increase in the sternal and parasternal fractures that are seen at post mortem. They are usually easily identified by their symmetrical, parasternal pattern and the relative lack of haemorrhage, which indicates their peri-mortem or post-mortem origin.

Penetrating injuries of the chest, whether the result of sharp force trauma (stab wounds) or gunshot wounds, may result in damage to any of the organs or vessels within the cavity. The effect of the penetration will depend mainly upon which organ(s) or vessel(s) are injured. The penetration of the chest wall will also result in the possibility of a pneumothorax.

Injury to the lungs will also result in the development of pneumothoraces, and damage to the blood vessels will result in haemorrhage, which may be confined to the soft tissues of the mediastinum or enter the pleural cavities. Haemorrhage from penetrating injuries to the chest will commonly remain concealed and it is not unusual to find several litres of blood within the chest cavity at post mortem. Alternatively, the haemorrhage will become apparent when the victim collapses, and the site of the injury then lies below the level of the blood in the chest cavity. This has important consequences for scene examination because the site of obvious blood loss may be some distance from the site of infliction of the injury.

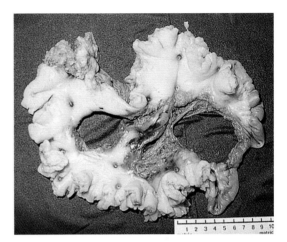
Figure 10.11 Lacerations of the mesentery, which resulted in fatal intra-abdominal haemorrhage following a blow from a knee.

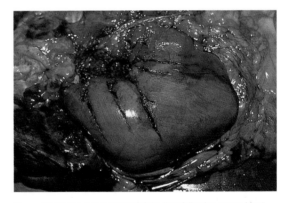
Figure 10.12 Extensive rupture of the liver following severe blunt abdominal trauma in a road traffic accident.

ABDOMEN

The anatomy of the abdominal cavity plays a major role in determining the type of injuries that are found. The vertebral column forms a strong midline vertical structure posteriorly, and blunt trauma, especially in the anterior/posterior direction, may result in compression of the organs lying in the midline against the vertebral column. This compressive injury may result in bruising or even rupture of the mesentery, bruising or even bisection of the duodenum or jejunum, rupture of the pancreas and laceration of the liver, especially the left lobe.

The forces required to cause these injuries in an adult must be considered to be severe and they are commonly found in road traffic accidents. It is unlikely

that a punch to the abdomen would cause more than simple bruising, except in very unusual circumstances, but kicks and stamps are commonly the cause of major intra-abdominal trauma. The kidneys and the spleen are attached only by their hila and are susceptible to rotational as well as direct trauma, and severe rotational forces may result in avulsion from their pedicles.

Abdominal injuries in children may have the same causes, but the forces required to cause them will be considerably reduced, and the slower compressive forces associated with squeezing of the abdomen during abuse may also result in the injuries described above.

Penetrating injuries to the abdomen can be the result of either gunshots or sharp force trauma. The effects of these injuries will depend almost entirely on the organs and vessels involved in the track of the projectiles. A penetrating injury to the aorta or inferior vena cava will result in severe haemorrhage and may produce rapid death. Peritonitis from a ruptured bowel or stomach will be immediately painful but may not, with adequate and prompt treatment, prove fatal.

Blunt trauma to the spleen is sometimes associated with delayed rupture leading to haemorrhage and possibly death some hours or even days after receipt of the injury. Pancreatic trauma may lead to the development of a pseudocyst, with little or no short-term or long-term sequelae.

Firearm and Explosive Injuries

Despite stringent legislation in the UK and elsewhere in the world, the use of firearms in criminal activities continues to increase. Weapons are becoming cheaper and easier to obtain as a result of the excessive and sometimes indiscriminate supply of arms and ammunition by governments and the acts and actions of national and international terrorist groups. The actions of these terrorist groups have also made some knowledge of explosive injuries essential for any practising forensic pathologist.

TYPES OF FIREARMS

There are two main types of firearm – those with smooth barrels, which fire groups of pellets or shot, and those with grooved or rifled barrels, which fire single projectiles or bullets. Both of these types of weapon rely upon the detonation of a solid propellant to produce the gases that propel the projectile(s). Air guns and air rifles form a separate group of weapons that rely upon compressed gas to propel the projectiles, and these weapons, together with the more unusual forms of projectile or firearm – the rubber bullet, stud guns and humane killers – are considered at the end of this section.

Shotguns

Shotguns, commonly used as sporting weapons, fire a large number of lead shot. The barrel, commonly 26–28 inches (66–71 cm) long, has a smooth internal surface. These guns may have one or two barrels; the double-barrelled weapons are arranged either side by side or 'over and under'. The muzzle is commonly slightly narrowed, which is known as a 'choke'. This 'choking' is used to control the shot pattern and the effect of the choking is to keep the shot together for longer.

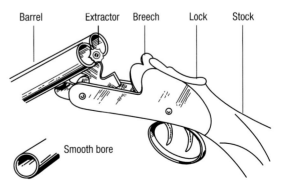

Figure 11.1 Diagram showing the detail of a twin-barrel shot gun – the gun is open (broken).

A shotgun is designed for use up to about 30–50 m and is unlikely to kill a man at this extreme range, although it may well cause serious and painful injuries. The length of the barrel makes handling and hiding difficult and so it is not uncommon for the barrels to be shortened – sawn off – for criminal activities. This shortening of the barrel has little effect on the properties of the gun and there is no doubt that shotguns can be devastating weapons at significant ranges.

The size of shotgun is usually given in relation to the 'gauge' or 'bore', which relates to the diameter of the barrel. The commonest size is the 12-bore or 12-gauge shotgun (which has a barrel diameter of 18.2 mm). The other popular shotgun has a barrel that is 0.410 inches (10.2 mm) in diameter and it is called, simply, a '410'.

The cartridges for shotguns consist of a metal base containing a central detonating cap, supporting a cardboard or plastic tube containing the propellant charge and a mass of lead shot, which rests on top of the propellant. The open end of the cartridge is closed by a thin disc, which is crimped into the end of the tube. The shot may be contained within a plastic bucket or there may be discs of felt, cork or cardboard acting as wads above and below the shot. The plastic containers open into a star shape in flight and may themselves cause injury.

The shot in the cartridges falls into one of two main groups – birdshot or buckshot – and the cartridges are numbered according to the size of the shot they contain. There are also cartridges that contain a single heavy projectile called a 'slug'. Occasionally, cartridges are tampered with and the loose shot is fused into a single mass. In some areas, especially developing countries or amongst rebels, homemade guns, sometimes called 'country guns', may be made from metal tubing with crude firing mechanisms. These weapons may be used to fire collections of debris such as nuts, bolts, wood-screws or metal shavings etc., and any wounds resulting from these weapons will obviously not comply with the usual descriptions.

Rifled weapons

These are weapons that fire one projectile at a time through a barrel that has a number of spiral grooves – usually between four and six and with a right-hand twist – cut into the interior of the barrel. The intervening projections, called 'lands', grip the bullet and

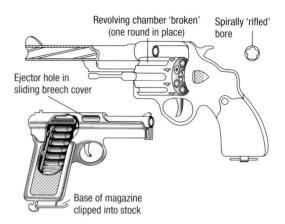

Figure 11.2 Diagrams of two types of handgun: a revolver (above) and a pistol (below). Note the rifling in the barrel.

impart the gyroscopic spin that assists in maintaining an accurate trajectory. Rifled weapons fall into three main groups – revolvers, 'automatic' pistols and rifles.

Revolvers and pistols are short-barrelled weapons and the difference between them is the method of presenting a bullet to the breech. In the revolver, a cylinder containing the bullets rotates under trigger pressure to line up a new cartridge with the trigger mechanism and the barrel. In a pistol, the forces generated by the firing of a round are harnessed using a spring mechanism to eject the spent cartridge case, load a fresh cartridge and reset the firing mechanism. The cartridges are usually stored in a clip contained within the butt of the weapon.

Rifles are long-barrelled weapons whose muzzle velocity and accuracy are much greater than those of the revolver or pistol. In older rifles, a bolt had to be moved manually to eject the spent cartridge case and bring a new round into the breech from a magazine. The gases generated from the discharge of the weapon are now used to perform the same tasks.

The ammunition for rifled weapons is also called a cartridge and comes in many sizes or calibres, usually measured from land to land. A cartridge is essentially a closed metal cylinder with the firing cap and propellant charge at one end and a single projectile – the bullet – clamped into the other. The bullet may be made of lead or lead alloy or it may have a lead core covered with a cupro-nickel, steel or other hard metal jacket. There may be a soft tip or an air space in the tip of the bullet, which is designed to distort and thus decelerate the bullet on impact. Some modern bullets have a small explosive charge in the tip for the same purpose.

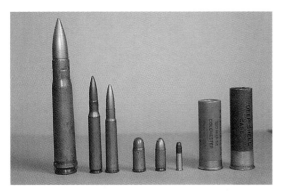

Figure 11.3 Various types of ammunition: From left to right: cannon shell, automatic rifle, bolt action rifle, revolver, pistol, .22 rifle, two 12-bore shotgun cartridges.

On a historical note, the term 'Dum-Dum bullets' relates to the .303 centrefire rifle cartridges with a hollow-point style bullet that were made at the British arsenal in Dum-Dum, India, in the late nineteenth century. The use of Dum-Dum and other expanding bullets was forbidden in wars between signatories of The Geneva Convention in 1864. This rule was reiterated by declarations of the Hague Conferences of 1899 and 1907. It should be noted that the restrictions apply to war only and that no restriction applies to the use of this type of bullet if war has not been formally declared.

Modern propellants consist of nitro-cellulose or other synthetic compounds prepared as small coloured flakes, discs or balls. The process of firing a bullet or shotgun cartridge is as follows. The firing pin strikes the primer cup and the primer compound explodes; small vents between the primer cup and the base of the cartridge case allow the flame of this detonation to spread to the propellant. The propellant burns rapidly, producing huge volumes of gas, which are further expanded by the very high temperatures of the ignition, and it is the pressure of this gas that propels the shot or bullet from the barrel.

The speed with which the projectile leaves the end of the barrel – the muzzle velocity – varies from a few hundred metres per second in a shotgun to a thousand or more in a high-velocity military weapon. The energy of the projectile is proportional to the speed at which it travels and is calculated from the kinetic energy ($\frac{1}{2}MV^2$) of the bullet, so higher muzzle velocities are considerably more effective at delivering energy to the target than larger bullets. The formation of wounds is related to the transfer of the energy of the bullet to the body tissues.

GUNSHOT WOUNDS

When any weapon is fired, smoke, flame and the gases of combustion will leave the barrel, together with portions of unburned, burning and burnt propellant. These contaminants will usually follow the projectile(s), but in some guns they may also precede them. The distance they will travel from the end of the muzzle is extremely variable, depending mainly on the type of weapon and the type of propellant. These contaminants also escape from small gaps around the breech and will soil hands or clothing that are close to the breech at the time of discharge.

Wounds from smooth-bore guns

The pellets are forced along the barrel by the gases of detonation and will leave the muzzle in a compact mass, which spreads out as it travels away from the gun. The shot describes a long, shallow cone with its apex close to the muzzle of the shotgun and the further along this cone the victim is situated, the larger the wound pattern will be.

A contact wound occurs when the muzzle is touching the skin and usually results in a circular entrance wound that is about the size of the muzzle. The wound edge will be regular and often has a clean-cut appearance with no individual pellet marks apparent. There will commonly be smoke soiling of at least some of the margin of the wound. There may be a narrow, circular rim of abrasion around some or all of the entrance wound, caused when the gases of the discharge enter through the wound and balloon the tissues upwards so that the skin is pressed against the muzzle. If the discharge was over an area supported by bone, the gases cannot disperse as quickly as they would in soft areas such as the abdomen, and the greater ballooning of the skin results in splits of the skin, which often have a radial pattern.

The wads or plastic cup will usually be recovered along the wound track. The tissues along the wound track will be blackened and the surrounding tissues are said to be pinker than normal as a result of the carbon monoxide contained within the discharge gases.

A close discharge, within a few centimetres of the surface, will also produce a wound with a similar appearance, but as there is now room for gas escape, there will be no muzzle mark. More smoke soiling can

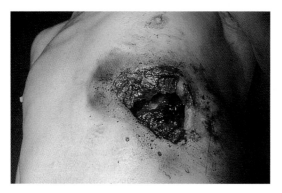

Figure 11.4 Close discharge of a 12-bore shotgun to the chest. There is a large hole, partly due to disruption by gas, and no evidence of pellet scatter is seen.

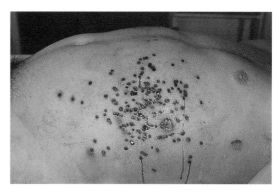

Figure 11.5 Medium-distance discharge of a 12-bore shotgun. The spread of the shot can be seen.

occur, and burning of skin with singeing and clubbing of melted hairs can be seen around the wound. There is also, very commonly, powder 'tattooing' of the skin around the entry wound. This tattooing is due to burnt and burning flakes of propellant causing tiny burns on the skin and cannot be washed off. Wads will commonly be found in the wound.

At intermediate ranges, between 20 cm and 1 m, there will be diminishing smoke soiling and burning of the skin, but powder tattooing may persist. The spread of shot will begin, first causing an irregular rim to the wound. Often called a 'rat-hole' in the USA because of the nibbled edges, the same appearance is called 'scalloping' in the UK. Separate injuries caused by the wads or plastic shot containers may be seen.

At a range of over 1 m, smoke damage and tattooing do not occur and injuries caused at longer ranges will depend upon the spread of the shot, which in turn is dependent upon the construction of the barrel. With a normal shotgun, satellite pellet holes begin to be seen around the main central wound at a range of about 2–3 m.

It is important to measure the spread of the shot so that if the weapon is recovered, test firings using identical ammunition can be performed to establish the range at which a particular spread of shot will occur. Estimates based on generalizations about the ratio of the diameter of this spread to the range should no longer be used.

At long ranges, such as 20–50 m, there is a uniform peppering of shot, and this is rarely fatal.

Shotguns rarely produce an exit wound when fired into the chest or abdomen, although single pellet exit

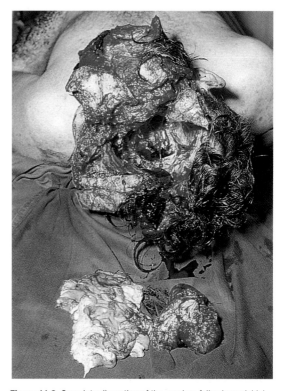

Figure 11.6 Complete disruption of the cranium following suicidal discharge of a shotgun in the mouth.

wounds can occasionally be seen. Exit wounds can be seen when a shotgun is fired into the head, neck or mouth. The exit wound in these cases may be a huge ragged aperture, especially in the head, where the skull may virtually explode with the gas pressure from a contact wound, ejecting part or even all of the brain from the cranial cavity.

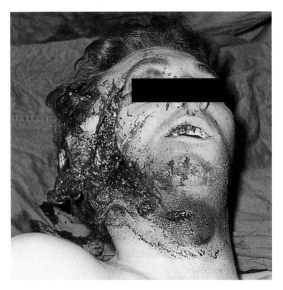

Figure 11.7 Close-range suicidal discharge of a shotgun below the chin. There is marked powder blackening of the chin and a ragged and irregular exit wound on the cheek.

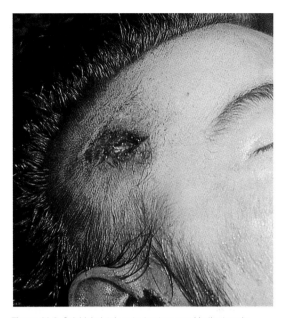

Figure 11.9 Suicidal pistol contact entry wound in the temple. The skin is burnt and split due to the gases of the discharge.

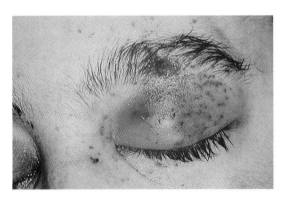

Figure 11.8 Pistol entry wound through the eyebrow with adjacent powder tattooing. The bruising of the eyelid is due to the fractured skull.

Wounds from rifled weapons

Bullets fired from rifled weapons will commonly cause both an entry and an exit wound. However, exceptions to this rule are numerous and many bullets are retained within the body because they did not possess enough energy to complete the passage.

Entrance wounds

Contact wounds from a rifled weapon are generally circular, unless over a bony area such as the head,

where splitting caused by the propellant gas is common. There may be a muzzle mark if the gun is pressed hard against the skin and a pattern may be imprinted from a fore-sight or self-loading mechanism. There may be slight escape of smoke with some local burning of skin and hair if the gun is not pressed tightly. Bruising around the entry wound is not uncommon.

At close range, up to about 20 cm, there will be some smoke soiling and powder burns, and skin and hair may be burnt, although this is very variable and depends upon both the gun and the ammunition used. The shape of the entry wound gives a guide to the angle that the gun made with that area of skin: a circular hole indicates that the discharge was at right angles to the skin, whereas an oval hole, perhaps with visible undercutting, indicates a more acute angle.

Examination of the entry wound will show that the skin is inverted; the defect is commonly slightly smaller than the diameter of the missile due to the elasticity of the skin. Very commonly, there is an 'abrasion collar' or 'abrasion rim' around the hole, which is caused by the friction, heating and dirt effect of the missile when it indents the skin during penetration. Bruising may or may not be associated with the wound.

Over 1 m or so, there can be no smoke soiling, burning or powder tattooing. At longer ranges (which may be up to several kilometres with a high-powered rifle), the entrance hole will have the same features of a round or oval defect with an abrasion collar. At extreme ranges, or following a ricochet, the gyroscopic stability of the bullet may be lost and the missile begins to wobble and even tumble, and this instability may well result in larger, more irregular wounds.

Exit wounds

The exit wound of a bullet is usually everted with split flaps, often resulting in a stellate appearance. There can be no burning, smoke or powder soiling. If the bullet has been distorted or fragmented or if it has fractured bone, the exit wound may be considerably larger and more irregular and those fragments of bullet or bone may be represented by multiple exit wounds.

Where skin is firmly supported, as by a belt, tight clothing or even leaning against a partition wall, the exit wound may be as small as the entrance and may fail to show the typical eversion. To increase the confusion, it may also show a rim of abrasion, although this is commonly broader than that of an entry wound.

The internal effects of bullets depend upon their kinetic energy. Low-velocity, low-energy missiles, such as shotgun pellets and some revolver bullets, cause simple mechanical disruption of the tissues by pushing them aside. High-velocity bullets cause far more

damage to the tissues as they transfer large amounts of energy, which results in the formation of a temporary cavity in the tissues. This cavity is many tens or hundreds of times larger than the calibre of the bullet itself. This cavitation is especially pronounced in dense organs such as liver and brain, but occurs in all tissues if the energy transfer is large enough and results in extensive tissue destruction away from the track itself.

AIR WEAPONS, UNUSUAL PROJECTILES AND OTHER WEAPONS

Air guns and rifles

Air weapons rely upon the force of compressed air to propel the projectile, usually a lead or steel pellet although darts and other projectiles may be used. There are three common ways in which the gas is compressed: the simplest employs the compression of a spring which, when released, moves a piston along a cylinder; more powerful weapons use repeated movements of a lever to pressurize an internal cylinder; and the third type has an internal cylinder which is 'charged' by connecting it to a pressurized external source. The barrel of an air weapon may or may not be rifled; the more powerful examples having similar rifling to ordinary handguns and rifles.

The energy of the projectile will depend mainly on the way in which the gas is compressed, the simple spring-driven weapons being low powered, while the more complex systems can propel projectiles with the same energy, and hence at approximately the same speed, as many ordinary handguns.

The injuries caused by the projectiles from air weapons will depend upon their design, but entry wounds from standard pellets are often indistinguishable from those caused by standard bullets in that they have a defect with an abrasion rim. The relatively low power of these weapons means that the pellet will seldom exit, but if it does so, a typical exit wound with everted margins will result.

Rubber and plastic bullets, stud guns and humane killers

In riot control, police may use plastic rounds fired from specially adapted guns. The purpose of these

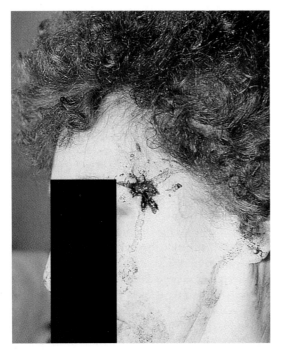

Figure 11.10 Typical stellate exit wound with everted margins.

weapons is to disable and discourage rioters but not to kill or seriously injure them. The plastic rounds are about 10 cm long, 3.5 cm in diameter and weigh about 130 g. They should not be fired at ranges less than about 20 m and should only be fired at the lower part of the body. Some deaths and many serious injuries, including fractures of skull, ribs and limbs and also eye damage and internal injuries, have occurred and these are usually associated with improper use. The mark left on the skin by a plastic round is usually distinctive.

Injuries and deaths from stud guns are well recorded. Stud guns are devices used in the building industry to fire steel pins into masonry or timber by means of a small explosive charge. They have been used for suicide and even homicide, but accidental injuries are more common. The skin injury often appears similar to many small-calibre entry wounds, although the finding of a nail will usually solve the diagnostic problem.

Humane killers are weapons used in abattoirs and by veterinary surgeons to kill animals. They may fire either a small-calibre bullet or a 'captive bolt', where a sliding steel pin is fired out for about 5 cm by an explosive charge. The skin injury will depend on the type of weapon used. These weapons have been used for both homicide and suicide, but accidental discharges are also recorded and may cause serious injury or death.

Bows and crossbows

These weapons fire arrows or bolts, which are shafts of wood or metal with a set of flights at the rear to maintain the trajectory of the projectile. The tips of these projectiles may have many shapes from the simple point to complex, often triangular, forms. The energy produced is extremely variable, depending on the construction of the weapon. The injuries caused depend on the energy of the projectile as well as on its construction. However, if the projectile has a simple pointed tip and if it has been removed from the body, the entry wounds can appear very similar to those caused by standard bullets, with a central defect and surrounding abrasion rim.

ACCIDENT, SUICIDE OR MURDER?

This is a major issue for the pathologist. Suicides must have wounds whose site and range are within the reach of the deceased's arm, unless some device has been used to reach the trigger. The weapon must be present at the scene, though it may be at a distance from the body because it may have been thrown away from the body by recoil or by movement of the individual if death was not immediate. Suicidal gunshot injuries are most commonly in the 'sites of election', which vary with the length of the weapon used. Both long-barrelled and short-barrelled weapons can be used in the mouth, below the chin, on the front of the neck, the centre of the forehead or, more rarely, the front of the chest over the heart. Discharges into the temples are almost unique to handguns and are usually on the side of the dominant hand, but this is not an absolute rule. People almost never shoot themselves in the eye or abdomen or in inaccessible sites such as the back. In Britain and many other countries, women rarely commit suicide with guns and are rarely involved in firearms accidents.

If suicide can be ruled out by the range of discharge, by absence of a weapon or by other features of the injury or the scene, a single gunshot injury could be either accident or homicide. Multiple firearm wounds, on the other hand, strongly suggest homicide. However, there have been a number of published reports of suicidal individuals who have fired repeatedly into themselves even when each wound is potentially fatal. The distinction between homicide, suicide and accident can sometimes be extremely difficult and a final conclusion can only be reached after a full police investigation.

The immediacy of death following receipt of injuries is discussed later (see Chapter 16) and it is as unwise to state that a gunshot wound, as with any other sort of injury, must have been immediately fatal. It is most likely that severe damage to the brain, heart, aorta and any number of other vital internal organs will lead to rapid collapse and death; however, this author has seen a case of long-term survival following a contact discharge of a shotgun into the head.

THE DOCTOR'S DUTY IN FIREARM INJURIES AND DEATHS

In the living, all efforts must be directed to saving life but, if at all possible, the treating doctor should make good notes of the original appearances of the injuries before any surgical cleaning or operative procedures are performed. Any missiles, foreign bodies such as wads, bullets or shot and any skin removed from the margin of a firearm wound during treatment should be carefully preserved for the police.

The same general rules apply to the post-mortem recovery of exhibits. The skin around the wounds may be swabbed for powder residues if this is considered to be necessary, but the retention of wounds themselves is no longer considered to be essential. Swabs of the hands of the victim should be taken. The pathologist must ensure that accurate drawings and measurements of the site, size and appearance of the wound are obtained and that distant and close-up photographs are taken of each injury with an appropriate scale in view.

In many countries, all firearm wounds, whether or not they are fatal, must be reported to the police. This applies in Northern Ireland (but not in mainland England), where the anti-terrorism legislation makes it compulsory for doctors to inform the police of any shooting or explosives injuries.

EXPLOSIVES

Terrorism and warfare lead to many deaths from explosive devices. In military bomb, shell and missile explosions, the release of energy may be so high that death and disruption from blast effects may occur over a wide area. In contrast, terrorist devices, unless they contain very large amounts of explosive, rarely compare with military effectiveness and thus the pure blast effects are far more limited. According to the inverse square law, the energy developed by an explosion decreases rapidly as the distance from the epicentre increases.

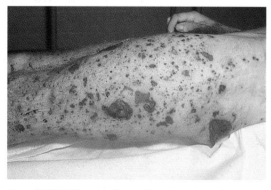

Figure 11.11 Multiple abrasions and lacerations due to flying debris projected by a terrorist bomb (courtesy of Professor T.K. Marshall, Belfast).

When an explosion occurs, the chemical interaction results in the generation of huge volumes of gas, which are further expanded by the great heat that is also generated. This sudden generation of gas causes a compression wave to sweep outwards; at the origin, this is at many times the speed of sound.

The pure blast effects can cause either physical fragmentation or disruption of the victim solely from the effects of the wave of high pressure and hot gases striking the body. A minimum pressure of about 700 kilopascals (100 lb/sq inch) is needed for tissue damage in humans. There will also be pressure effects upon the viscera and these effects are far more damaging where there is an air/fluid interface, such as in the air passages, the lungs and the gut. Ruptures and haemorrhage of these areas represent the classical blast lesion.

Dangerous though the effect of blast is, many more casualties, fatal and otherwise, are caused by secondary effects of explosive devices, especially in the lower-powered terrorist bombs. These secondary effects include:

- burns – directly from the near effects of the explosion and secondarily from fires started by the bomb;
- missile injuries from parts of the bomb casing or shrapnel or from adjacent objects;
- peppering by small fragments of debris and dust propelled by the explosion;
- all types of injury due to collapse of structures caused by the explosion;
- injuries and death from vehicular damage or destruction, such as decompression, fire and ground impact of bombed aircraft and crash damage to cars, trucks, buses etc.

Examination of either the living or the dead following an explosion is essential, with careful documentation of the sites and sizes of the abrasions, bruises, lacerations, burns and any other injuries.

If a near or massive explosion disrupts one or more bodies, identification of the fragments is essential, not least to determine how many victims were killed. This task can be extremely difficult and resembles the response to a mass disaster such as an air crash, in which many bodies may be severely disrupted and burnt. The difference is that, following a terrorist bombing, the pathologist has an additional task, which is to assist in the identification and recovery of material that might have formed part of the bomb.

Transportation Injuries

Every form of transport is associated with a risk and, as the speed of transport increases, particularly as mechanization is involved, the risks of an accident are increased and the effects of an accident are magnified.

ROAD TRAFFIC INJURIES

Those injured by accidents on the road can be divided into three broad groups: pedestrians, cyclists (pedal or motor) and the drivers and passengers of vehicles. Of these three broad groups, it is the pedestrians that are most often injured, although the proportion of pedestrian victims in the overall statistics varies greatly according to the traffic patterns of different countries. It is perhaps self-evident that where there is greater mingling of motor transport and pedestrians there is also a greater risk of injury to the pedestrian. In 1998, 85 per cent of all road deaths in the world occurred in developing countries, where death rates of nearly 30 per 100 000 per annum are common; high-income countries generally have death rates of less than 5 per 100 000 per annum.

Pedestrians

Pedestrians struck by motor vehicles suffer injuries from direct contact with the vehicle (primary injuries) or from contact with other objects or the ground after the contact with the vehicle (secondary injuries).

The primary injuries can often form recognizable patterns. When an adult is hit by the front of a car, the front bumper (fender) usually strikes the victim at about knee level. The exact point of contact, whether on the front, side or back of the leg(s), will depend on the orientation of the victim. There are often additional primary injury sites on the thigh, hip or pelvis due to contact with the edge of the bonnet (hood). At low speeds (e.g. 20 kph/12 mph), the victim will commonly be thrown off the bonnet either forwards or to one side. Between 20 and 60 kph (12–36 mph), the victim will be tipped onto the bonnet (hood) and the head may strike the windscreen or the metal frame that surrounds it. At higher speeds (60–100 kph/ 36–60 mph), the victim may be projected (scooped) up into the air; sometimes they will pass completely over the vehicle and will avoid hitting the windscreen and other points on the vehicle.

The secondary injuries are often more serious and potentially lethal than the primary injuries. The constellation of these secondary injuries is wide; they vary from the 'brush abrasions' caused by skidding across the surface of the road to fractures of the skull or axial skeleton caused by direct contact with a surface, to fractures of the spine, which can be caused by hyperflexion or extension. It is important to remember that the external

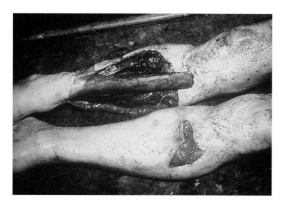

Figure 12.1 Compound fracture of the right leg and laceration of the left knee in a pedestrian struck by a car. It is most likely that the vehicle struck the right leg.

injuries are seldom of themselves lethal; it is their association with internal injuries that is important.

Even without fractures of the skull, brain damage is frequent and is caused when the moving head of the victim is suddenly stopped on impact; more diffuse damage to axons may be caused by the rotational or shearing forces acting upon the brain inside the rapidly moving head. Fractures of the spine, especially in the cervical and thoracic segments, may lead to cord damage. Fractures of the limbs are common but, apart from those of the legs that are associated with the primary impact sites, they are somewhat unpredictable because of the random flailing of the limbs.

Where the vehicle is relatively larger than the victim – adults impacted by larger vehicles and children impacted by cars – the point of contact is higher up the victim and it is likely that the victim will make contact with more of the front of the vehicle. This pattern of contact will be reflected in the resulting primary injuries to the pelvis, abdomen, chest and head. It is more likely that the victim will be projected along the line of travel of the vehicle, which may increase the risk of 'running-over' injuries.

'Running-over' injuries are relatively unusual and the effects are variable, depending on the area of the body involved, the weight of the vehicle and the surface area of the contact. The skull may be disrupted and the brain externalized; internal organs may be ruptured and there may be fractures of the spine. Compression of the chest may result in multiple rib fractures, causing a 'flail chest'. The rotation of the wheel may strip off large areas of skin and subcutaneous tissue; this is called a 'flaying injury'.

Car occupants

Most impacts involve the front or the front corners of the vehicle and approximately 80 per cent of impacts are against either another vehicle or a stationary object. This type of impact rapidly decelerates the vehicle. Less commonly, the vehicle is hit from behind, causing an 'acceleration' impact. The least common impacts are side impacts and 'roll-overs'.

In the common deceleration situation without restraint, the front-seat occupants move forwards as the vehicle decelerates around them and they strike the vehicle structures that are in front of them. In general terms, the following may be expected in an unrestrained impact.

- The face and head hit the windscreen glass, frame or side-pillars, causing fractures to the skull and cervical spine and also brain injury.
- The chest and abdomen contact the fascia or the steering wheel, causing rib, sternal, heart and liver damage.
- The momentum of the heart within the thorax, perhaps aided by hyperflexion, may tear the aorta at the termination of the descending part of the arch, at the point where the vessel becomes attached to the vertebral column.
- The legs of the passenger are thrown forwards and the knees may strike the parcel shelf, causing fractures.
- The legs of the driver, which are commonly braced on the brake and clutch pedals, may transmit the force of impact along the tibia and femur to the pelvis. All of these bones may be fractured or dislocated.
- On the rebound from these impacts, the heavy head may swing violently backwards and cause injury to the cervical or thoracic spine.
- The occupants of the car may be ejected out of the vehicle through the windscreen, increasing the risks of secondary injuries or running over.

The unrestrained rear-seat passenger is also liable to injury through either deceleration or acceleration. The injuries, in general, may not be as severe as those caused to the front-seat occupants. In a deceleration impact, the rear-seat passengers will be thrown against the backs of the front seats and may impact the front-seat occupants. They may be projected over the front seat to hit the windscreen and even be thrown out through the windscreen. The introduction of seat belts has dramatically reduced the number and severity of injuries to car occupants.

THE FUNCTION OF SEAT BELTS

The introduction of the mandatory use of seat belts has had a profound effect on road traffic fatality rates in the UK. Seat belts have undergone numerous design changes: the simple lap strap, such as that used for aircraft passengers, is of little value in cars and may even be dangerous; the full double shoulder harness used in light aircraft and gliders provides excellent protection but is not acceptable to car users; and the combination of a lap strap and a diagonal shoulder strap was introduced as a satisfactory compromise between effectiveness and social acceptability. To be effective, they have to be worn correctly and any alteration in their fixing, structure or use rapidly degrades their value.

A seat belt that is correctly installed and correctly worn acts in the following ways.

- It spreads the deceleration forces over the whole area of contact of the straps against the body surface so that the force per unit area of the body is reduced.
- It is designed to stretch during deceleration and some belts have a specific area for this to occur. This stretching slightly extends the time of deceleration and reduces the force per unit time.
- It restrains the body during deceleration, keeping it away from the windscreen, steering wheel and other frontal obstructions, thus protecting the head.
- It prevents ejection into the road through burst doors or windows, which used to be a common cause of severe injury and death.

AIR BAGS

The development of air bags was an attempt to aid the protection of all car occupants but in particular those who did not wear seat belts. The concept of an air bag is simple: a rapidly deploying soft method of restraint that is only present when required.

The deployment of an air bag relies upon the explosive production of gas, usually from the detonation of a pellet commonly made of sodium azide. For the deployment to be timed correctly, the deceleration of the vehicle following impact needs to be sensed and the detonation of the pellet completed in microseconds so that the bag is correctly inflated at the time the occupant of the car is beginning to move towards the framework of the vehicle.

Air bags are designed to provide protection to the average adult in the front of the car and this protection depends upon the occupant responding in an 'average' fashion; the explosive nature of the deployment of air bag has, on rare occasions, resulted in injuries to the occupants of vehicles. Those especially at risk are drivers of short stature who have to sit nearer the steering wheel than normal.

At particular risk are babies who are placed on the front passenger seat in a rear-facing baby seat that is held in place by the seat belt. The back of the baby seat may lie within the range of the bag when it is maximally expanded, and fatalities have been recorded following relatively minor vehicle impacts when the air bag has struck the back of the baby seat. The passenger airbag should be deactivated when a baby is placed on the front passenger seat.

Motor cycle and pedal cycle injuries

Most injuries to motor cyclists are due to falling from the machine onto the roadway. Many of the injuries can be reduced or prevented by the wearing of suitable protective clothing and a crash helmet. Abrasions due to contact with the road surface are almost universal following an accident at speed, and injuries to the limbs and to the chest and spine occur very commonly due to contact with other objects or vehicles, entanglement with the motor bike or direct contact with the road. Despite the introduction of the mandatory wearing of crash helmets in the UK, head injuries are still a common cause of morbidity and mortality. A more unique injury occurs from 'tail-gating', where the motorcyclist drives under the rear of a truck, causing severe head injuries or even decapitation. This injury has been reduced by the presence of bars at the sides and rear of trucks to prevent both bikes and cars passing under the vehicle.

Injuries associated with pedal cycles are very common due to the large numbers of cycles in use. Most injuries associated with cycles tend to be of mild or moderate severity due to their low speeds. However, impact by vehicles can result in severe and fatal injuries. Secondary injuries, especially head and chest

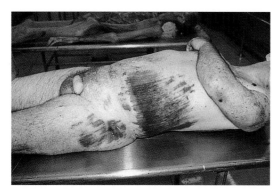

Figure 12.2 Extensive 'brush' abrasion of the left flank in a motor cyclist thrown across a rough surface.

damage, are common when cyclists fall from their relatively high riding position on such an inherently unstable machine.

THE MEDICAL EXAMINATION OF VICTIMS OF ROAD TRAFFIC ACCIDENTS

A doctor may be called, either to treat living victims or to examine fatal casualties of road traffic accidents. If the victim is still alive, the first duty of any doctor is to assist that individual to the best of his ability. Anyone involved in the aftermath of an accident may be called to an enquiry or court hearing, and civil actions for negligence may arise and insurance claims may be pursued. Any doctor should make and keep a note of treatment given, even if they have done so as a 'Good Samaritan' act by the side of the road.

The victim should be carefully examined externally and all injuries recorded (see Chapter 9). Injuries should be measured with a ruler and patterns should be noted with great care. Tyre marks, often in the form of abrasions or intradermal bruising, may be present on the skin of both living and dead victims and so a photograph or accurate, measured drawing may be of great value in helping to identify a 'hit-and-run' car or truck. For pedestrian victims, the distance above the heel of the upper and lower margins of the major injuries should be measured because these heights can be correlated with the height of the bumper (fender), the bonnet and other features on a suspect vehicle.

In countries where there is an established forensic science service, examination of the clothing may reasonably be left to the scientists, but if no such service

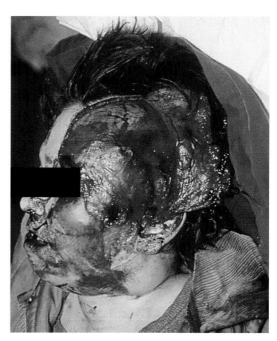

Figure 12.3 A 'flaying' injury due to a rotating wheel crossing the left side of the face.

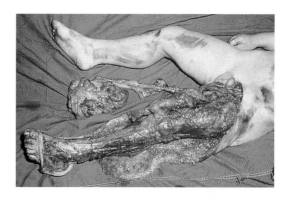

Figure 12.4 Pedestrian leg injury from a rotating wheel resulting in 'flaying' of the skin.

exists or if it is not available to the doctor, the clothing should be examined for tears, soiling by oil, grease or road dirt etc. and any broken glass, paint flakes, rust or foreign material should be carefully documented and preserved for the police.

The possibility that alcohol or drugs have contributed to the accident should always be considered and samples retained for analysis at post mortem. The living victim must give consent to the taking of samples for such a test or for the testing of samples taken for other purposes (see Chapter 23).

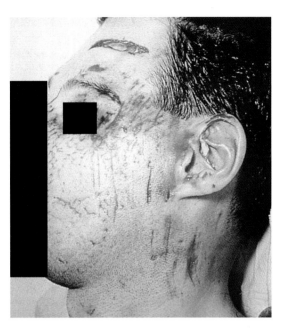

Figure 12.5 Facial injuries on a driver who did not wear a seat belt.

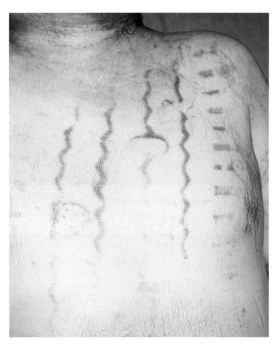

Figure 12.7 Intradermal bruising reflecting the tyre tread pattern. Note the bruising is of the 'valleys' and not the 'hills' in the tread.

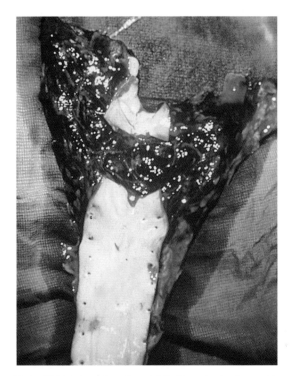

Figure 12.6 Ruptured thoracic aorta following a deceleration impact. The rupture is at the termination of the arch and has resulted in extensive haemorrhage.

RAILWAY INJURIES

These are most common in countries with a large railway network, such as India and China, and where railroad crossings are unprotected. Although mass disasters such as the derailment of a train occasionally lead to large numbers of casualties, most deaths and injuries occur as an aggregation of numerous individual incidents, most of which are accidents, as at level crossings or due to children playing on the line. There is also an appreciable number of suicides in all countries.

Medically, there is nothing specific about railway injuries except the frequency of very severe mutilation. The body may be severed into many pieces and soiled by axle grease and dirt from the wheels and track. Where passengers fall from a train at speed, multiple injuries due to repeated impacts and rolling may be seen, often with multiple abrasions from contact with the coarse gravel of the line ballast.

Suicides on railways fall into two main groups: those that lie on the track (sometimes placing their neck across a rail so that they are beheaded) and those that jump in front of a moving train from a platform, bridge or other structure near to the track. Jumping

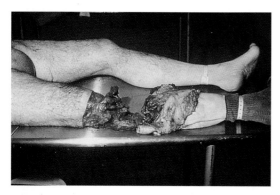

Figure 12.8 Clean amputation of the leg from a railway wheel.

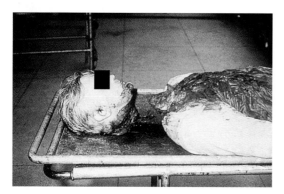

Figure 12.9 Suicidal decapitation on a railway line. Note the soiling of the neck margin.

from a moving train is much less common. The injuries present will depend on the exact events, but they are usually extensive and severe when there has been contact with a moving train, although they may be localized with black soiling at the crushed decapitation or amputation site if the individual has lain across the track.

A careful search for unusual injuries and for a vital response to the severe blunt force injuries should be made, as there have been occasions when the victim of a homicide has been placed onto the rail track in an attempt to conceal the true cause of death.

Railway workers may be injured or killed by falling under or by being struck by moving rolling stock or by being trapped between the buffers of two trucks whilst uncoupling or coupling the rolling stock. The injuries associated with the squeezing between rolling stock are often those of a 'flail chest', with or without evidence of 'traumatic asphyxia'.

On electrified lines, an additional cause of suicidal or accidental injury or death is present in the form of electric shock from either a live rail or overhead power lines. The voltage in these circuits is high, often in region of 600 volts. Death is rapid and often associated with severe burns at the points of contact or earthing.

AIRCRAFT FATALITIES

Aviation incidents can be divided into two main groups: those that involve the crew and the large numbers of passengers of a modern, commercial airliner, and those that involve the occupants of small, relatively slow, light aircraft.

Large aircraft are pressurized and if the integrity of the cabin is breached, there can be rapid decompression and the passengers may suffer barotrauma. If the defect in the cabin is large enough, victims may be sucked out and fall to their death. When an aircraft hits the ground, the results will naturally depend on the rapidity of transfer of the forces and this is dependent on the speed of the aircraft and the angle of impact. If the forces are very severe, all passengers may be killed by pure deceleration injury and by multiple trauma due to loss of integrity of the fuselage.

In lesser impacts, the results may be similar to those of motor vehicle crashes, although the forces are usually greater and the injuries sustained are proportionately more severe. The usual lap-strap seat belt offers little protection in anything but the most minor accident. Fire is one of the greatest hazards in air crashes and accounts for many deaths.

In light aircraft crashes, the velocity, and hence the forces, may be less than in large commercial aircraft, but they are still often fatal. The investigation of air accidents is a task for specialist medical personnel, who are often available from the national air force or from a civil authority. There should always be a full autopsy on the pilot or suspected pilot, with full microscopic and toxicological examination to exclude natural disease, drugs and alcohol.

MASS DISASTERS AND THE DOCTOR

For the non-specialist doctor at the scene of a mass disaster of any kind, the first consideration is, of course, the treatment of casualties, which may involve taking difficult ethical decisions about triage. The World Medical Association published a useful statement about the medical ethics in disasters at its assembly in 1994. Among other things, the statement recommends that triage should be entrusted to an authorized and experienced physician, who should be accompanied by competent staff. It also indicates that triage is not a 'one-off' review and that regular reassessments must be made as cases may evolve and change category.

Victims can be divided into five main groups:

1 those who can be saved and whose lives are in immediate danger;
2 those whose lives are not in immediate danger but who are in need or urgent but not immediate medical care;
3 those who have minor injuries only and who can be treated later or by unskilled personnel;
4 those who have been psychologically traumatized and who need reassurance and/or sedation if acutely disturbed;
5 those whose condition exceeds the available therapeutic resources and who have suffered from such extremely severe injuries of whatever type that they cannot be saved in the specific circumstances of that time and place: these victims can be termed 'beyond emergency care'.

The World Medical Association statement makes it clear that to abandon an injured person on account of the priorities dictated by the disaster situation cannot be considered to be a failure, but that it is justified because these decisions are intended to save the maximum number of victims – the greatest good to the greatest number.

The investigation of the causes of death and the causes of the incident (such as a bomb) and the identification of the dead are specialist operations involving mortuary accommodation, pathology, dentistry, the police and the usual state agencies responsible for sudden death; in England and Wales this is the coroner. A team of pathologists, assisted by police officers and mortuary staff and backed up by dental and radiological facilities, inspects every body and records all clothing, jewellery and personal belongings still attached to the bodies. The body or body part is then carefully examined for every aspect of identity, including sex, race, height, age and personal characteristics. All these details are recorded on standard forms and charts and the information is sent back to the identification teams, which can compare this information from the bodies with the information obtained from relatives, friends etc. An autopsy is performed to determine the cause of death, to retrieve any foreign objects that, for example, may be related to an explosive device, and to seek any further identifying factors, such as operation sites, prostheses etc.

Chapter thirteen

Asphyxia

Suffocation	Café coronary	**Ligature strangulation**
Smothering	**Pressure on the neck**	**Hanging**
Gagging	**'Vagal inhibition' or reflex cardiac arrest**	**The sexual asphyxias**
Choking	**Manual strangulation**	**Traumatic asphyxia**

The literal translation of the word asphyxia from the Greek means 'absence of pulse' and how this word has come to denote the effects of the lack of oxygen is not clear, but the word asphyxia is now commonly used to describe a range of conditions for which the lack of oxygen – whether it is partial (hypoxia) or complete (anoxia) – is considered to be the cause.

In the forensic context, asphyxia is usually obstructive in nature, where some physical barrier prevents access of air to the lungs; this obstruction can occur at any point from the nose and mouth to the alveolar membranes. Other conditions in which the body cannot gain sufficient oxygen may occur without any obstruction to the air passages. Given the many possible causes for this lack of sufficient oxygen to the cells of the body, it is not surprising that the clinical and pathological features of the many different types of 'asphyxia' are very varied.

The 'classical' features of asphyxia are found where the air passages are obstructed by pressure applied to the neck or to the chest and where there has been a struggle to breathe. The classical features of 'asphyxia' are:

1 congestion of the face;
2 oedema of the face;
3 cyanosis (blueness) of the skin of the face;
4 petechial haemorrhages in the skin of the face and the eyes.

A fifth feature – increased fluidity of the blood – is now not accepted. The other four features, although not diagnostic, are important and are considered below.

Congestion is the red appearance of the skin of the face and head. It is due to the filling of the venous system when compression of the neck or some other obstruction prevents venous return to the heart.

Oedema is the swelling of the tissues due to transudation of fluid from the veins caused by the increased venous pressure as a result of obstruction of venous return to the heart.

Cyanosis is the blue colour imparted to the skin by the presence of deoxygenated blood in the congested venous system and, possibly, in the arterial system.

Petechial haemorrhages (petechiae) are tiny, pinpoint haemorrhages, most commonly seen in the skin of the head and face and especially in the lax tissues of the eyelids. They are also seen in the conjunctivae and sclera of the eye. They are due to leakage of blood from small venules as a result of the raised pressure in the venous system. The theory that they are caused, at least in part, by hypoxia of the blood vessel walls is not supported by research. They are not diagnostic of asphyxia because they can appear instantaneously in the face and eyes following a violent episode of sneezing or coughing.

Petechiae on the pleural surface of the lungs, the epicardium and the thymus in children, are the true

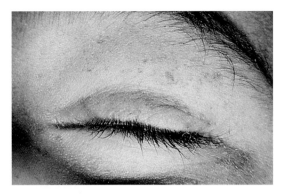

Figure 13.1 Petechial haemorrhages on the eyelid in a case of manual strangulation.

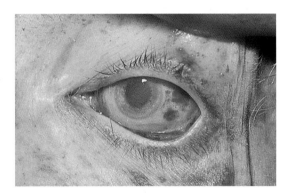

Figure 13.2 Conjunctival haemorrhages in manual strangulation.

Table 13.1 'Asphyxial' Conditions

Underlying cause of death	Name
Lack of oxygen in the inspired air	Suffocation
Blockage of the external orifices	Suffocation/smothering
Blockage of the internal airways by obstruction	Gagging/choking
Blockage of the internal airways by external pressure	Strangulation/hanging
Restriction of chest movement	Traumatic asphyxia
Failure of oxygen transportation	For example CO poisoning
Failure of oxygen utilization	For example cyanide poisoning

3 Loss of consciousness and possible convulsions; evacuation of bladder and vomiting.

4 Reduction in the depth and frequency of respiration; irreversible brain damage begins; the pupils dilate and death ensues.

At any stage through this progression, death may occur suddenly from cardiac arrest.

The classification and nomenclature of the various 'asphyxial' conditions are imprecise, adding to the confusion over this group of deaths (Table 13.1).

SUFFOCATION

Situations in which accumulations of irrespirable gases occur are commonly industrial or agricultural; they may be found in the deep tanks of ships where rust formation has removed oxygen, in farm silos containing grain, or in deep wells in chalk where carbon dioxide has accumulated. The individual entering these situations without protective equipment will be rendered unconscious extremely quickly and will die rapidly unless removed from the hypoxic environment. In all these situations, asphyxial signs may be minimal as collapse and death may be so rapid.

Rapid deaths are also reported when a plastic bag is placed over the head, either as a deliberate suicidal act or accidentally by children. Typically, no 'classic signs' are seen and the face is usually pale when the bag is removed. The bag need not be tied around the neck to be effective.

Tardieu spots described in the nineteenth century by Professor Ambroise Tardieu, who thought, incorrectly, that they were an infallible hallmark of asphyxia. A few petechial haemorrhages can be seen on the surface of the lungs, heart etc. in many other conditions, but of particular importance is the finding that approximately 70 per cent of 'cot deaths' (SIDS) have them and they are often large and numerous in this situation. It is important that these petechiae are not interpreted as evidence of external respiratory obstruction.

A person with obstructed air entry will show various phases of distress and physical signs, the exact timing and the sequence of events will be very variable, but they may progress as listed below.

1 Increased efforts to breathe, facial congestion and the onset of cyanosis.

2 Deep, laboured respirations or attempts at respiration with a heaving chest; deepening congestion and cyanosis; the appearance of petechiae if venous return is impaired.

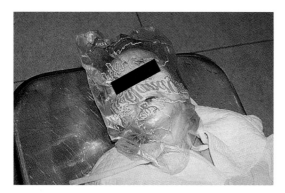

Figure 13.3 'Exit' suicide with a plastic bag. The face is usually pale and devoid of asphyxial signs.

SMOTHERING

Smothering with a pillow or other object (including a hand) pressed over the nose and mouth will only very rarely cause any petechiae, any significant cyanosis or congestion unless the victim struggles and fights for breath against the obstructed airways. Smothering may be virtually impossible to diagnose if it is applied to those who cannot or do not resist – the old, the infirm or the very young. If the victim does struggle, there may be bruises and abrasions to the face, on the lips or inside the mouth (where lips are pressed against teeth).

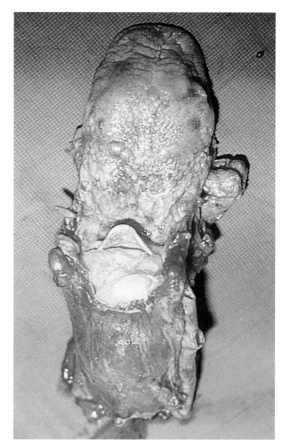

Figure 13.4 Impaction of food in the larynx – café coronary.

GAGGING

The air passages may be obstructed when a cloth or soft object is pushed into the mouth, or placed across the mouth, often during a robbery when the victim is tied up and the cloth is used to ensure their silence. At first, breathing can take place via the nose, but as time goes on, nasal mucus and oedema close the posterior nares and progressive asphyxia develops.

CHOKING

Manual strangulation is occasionally referred to as 'choking', but this is incorrect. The term choking should be applied to the internal obstruction of the upper air passages by an object or substance impacted in the pharynx or larynx. Choking is, most commonly,

accidental and the causes include dentures in adults and inhaled objects such as small toys, balls etc. in children. In medical practice there are risks associated with individuals who are sedated or anaesthetized, when objects such as extracted teeth or blood from dental or ENT operations may occlude the airway without provoking the normal reflex of coughing. Obstruction commonly leads to respiratory distress with congestion and cyanosis of the head and face.

Café coronary

Perhaps the commonest cause of choking is the entry of food into the air passages. If food enters the larynx during swallowing, it usually causes gross 'choking symptoms' of coughing, distress and cyanosis, which can be fatal unless the obstruction is cleared by coughing or some rapid treatment is offered. However, if the piece of food is large enough to occlude the larynx completely, it will prevent not only breathing but also speech and coughing. The individual may die silently and quickly, the cause of death remaining hidden until the autopsy. This is the so-called café coronary.

The airways are normally protected from the entry of food or vomit by powerful reflexes, and anything that can reduce or eliminate those reflexes will render the individual at greater risk, for example acute alcohol intoxication, depressant drugs, anaesthetics or many kinds of neurological disease. The acid nature of vomit will have an inflammatory effect in addition to the simple mechanical obstruction of the material. However, the finding of stomach contents in the larynx, trachea and bronchi is common at autopsy and it is not safe to conclude, on autopsy findings alone, that death was due to aspiration of stomach contents. The presence of vomit in the airways may be an agonal or post-mortem artefact. Research has shown that when barium is placed in the stomach after death, x-rays commonly reveal barium in the bronchial tree following routine post-mortem handling of the body.

PRESSURE ON THE NECK

Three forms of pressure on the neck are of prime forensic importance, namely, manual strangulation, ligature strangulation and hanging. In all of these, death may be relatively slow, with the formation of the 'classic' asphyxial signs of cyanosis, congestion, oedema and petechiae, or death may be rapid or even instantaneous due to sudden cardiac arrest, in which case a pale face with no cyanosis, congestion or petechiae may be observed.

When pressure is applied to the neck, the effects listed below may occur. However, the precise events in any single case will depend upon the method used, the site(s) of pressure and the force with which the pressure is applied.

- Obstruction of the jugular veins, causing impaired venous return of blood from the head to the heart. This leads to cyanosis, congestion, petechiae etc.
- Obstruction of the carotid arteries, which if severe, causes cerebral ischaemia.
- Stimulation of the baroceptor nerve endings in the carotid sinuses, which lie in the internal carotid

artery just above the carotid bifurcation, leading to effects on the heart through the vagus nerve.
- Elevation of the larynx and tongue, closing the airway at pharyngeal level. It is difficult to occlude the airway at laryngeal or tracheal level, due to the rigidity of the strong cartilages, unless extreme pressure is applied.

'VAGAL INHIBITION' OR REFLEX CARDIAC ARREST

Reflex cardiac arrest is a very real and common occurrence, especially when associated with pressure on the neck. Stimulation of the carotid sinus baroceptors causes impulses to pass via Hering's nerve to the afferent fibres of the glossopharyngeal nerves (9th cranial nerve); these in turn link in the brainstem to the nucleus of the 10th cranial nerve (vagus). Parasympathetic efferent impulses then descend to the heart via the cardiac branches of the vagus nerve. Stimulation of these fibres causes a profound bradycardia, which can occasionally amount to total cardiac arrest. This effect is often known as 'vagal inhibition' and, although the term is often overused, sometimes in inappropriate circumstances, it remains a useful term, which the forensic practitioner should be sure to use in a precise manner.

It is well accepted that in some cases of strangulation, and in rather more cases of hanging, the sudden application of pressure onto one or other carotid sinus can initiate rapid death, through the vagally mediated cardiac bradycardia described above, before any congestive or petechial signs have time to appear – and so the victim dies with a pale face and no petechiae.

The length of time that pressure must be maintained to produce congestion and petechiae in a living victim is matter of controversy, but it is generally (although not universally) agreed that a minimum of 15–30 seconds is required. It is concluded from this that the absence of these features indicates that death must have supervened within that length of time. This may be of legal significance in assessing the determination with which an assailant held on to his victim. However, it is clear that any amount of pressure applied to the neck for any amount of time can result in death and so there can be no entirely 'safe' way to hold or compress the neck.

MANUAL STRANGULATION

This is a relatively common mode of homicide used by a man against a woman or a child and it is sometimes associated with a sexual attack. It is relatively unusual for a man to throttle another man, and women rarely strangle, except as a means of infanticide.

Manual strangulation may be performed by one or both hands, from the front or the back. The hand or hands may be applied, loosened and reapplied over and over again during the course of an attack, making it extremely difficult to interpret the injuries on the neck. The external signs are abrasions and bruises on the front and sides of the neck and there are commonly injuries at each side of the laryngeal prominence and just below the jaw line. The injuries may be much more widespread, even extending onto the upper part of the sternal area. Typical fingertip bruising may be seen, which consists of disc-shaped or oval-shaped bruises about 0.5–1 cm in size.

There may also be linear abrasions or scratches from fingernails. If these are from the assailant, they are commonly vertically orientated. However, victims may also mark their own necks while trying to prise away the strangling fingers; these linear marks commonly lie close to areas of bruising and are often horizontally orientated.

When pressure has been more prolonged, the classic signs of venous obstruction will be seen, with cyanosis, oedema and congestion of the face together with showers of petechiae in the eyes and face and sometimes bleeding from nose and ears. If pressure has been sustained, congestion and cyanosis of the neck structures will also be seen and there may be petechiae on the epiglottis and visceral pleura.

Caution must be used in interpreting bleeding into the posterior neck tissues, as this is a very common artefact in all types of autopsy. When strangulation or hanging is suspected from the circumstances or from the external appearances, it is important that the dissection of the neck should not be carried out until the great veins in the thorax have been opened, which allows the blood from the head and neck to drain and for the dissection to be performed in a relatively bloodless field.

The larynx is commonly damaged during manual strangulation and the most vulnerable structures are the superior horns of the thyroid cartilage, which may be fractured on one or both sides. The hyoid bone is much less often injured, but when it is injured, one or both of the greater horns may be broken. These fractures of the laryngeal cartilages rarely occur in children or young people as the cartilage is pliable, but the calcification and ossification of increasing age render these cartilages more brittle and vulnerable to trauma. Very rarely, the cricoid cartilage is fractured and the main plate of the thyroid cartilage can be split; these features are indicative of the application of severe levels of localized force and are more consistent with a forceful punch or a kick than simple manual strangulation.

Surprisingly, there have been a few, rather doubtful, reports of manual self-strangulation. Obviously, these must have caused death through sudden vagal inhibition, but it is difficult to understand how an act with such an unpredictable outcome could be considered suicidal.

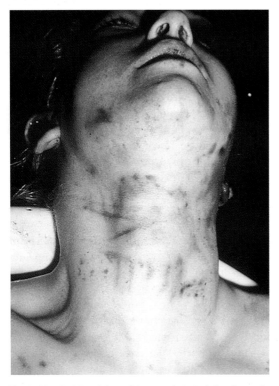

Figure 13.5 Bruising of the neck in manual strangulation. Some of the bruises are due to the victim trying to release the grip of the assailant.

LIGATURE STRANGULATION

Here, a constricting band is tightened around the neck, which usually results in marked congestion and cyanosis and extensive petechiae in the face. All types of ligature can be used: rope, wire, string, electric and telephone cable, scarves, stockings, pieces of cloth etc.

The mark on the neck will usually reflect the material used for the ligature: if a wire or thin cord was used, the mark will usually be clear-cut and deep with sharply defined edges. If a soft fabric is pulled taut, it will commonly fold into a series of firm ridges or bands that may produce interlacing deeper areas of bruising on the neck of the victim, which can suggest the use of a narrow ligature.

The ligature mark is a vital piece of evidence, especially when the killer has taken away the actual ligature. The mark on the neck may reproduce the pattern of the object, such as spiral or plaited weave, and the width of the mark can sometimes give a clue as to the size of the ligature. If the ligature has been left on after death or if sliding friction has occurred, the mark on the neck will be a brownish, dried leathery band, sometimes deeply sunk into the tissues. There may be a red flare of 'vital reaction' on either side of the ligature mark. The position of the mark is usually just above the laryngeal prominence. The mark usually goes around the whole circumference of the neck, but it need not necessarily do so if clothing or hair has become interposed between the ligature and the skin. It is important to look for the site of a crossover of the ligature mark or for any knots that may be present. These may be at the front, back or the sides and will give some idea of the relative position of the perpetrator. The ligature mark may lie horizontally or at an angle, but, crucially, it will not have a suspension point, which is commonly found in many hangings.

Occasionally, a ligature mark may lie only across the front of the neck, which indicates that the assailant either pressed from the front or pulled from the back using a cord stretched between two hands. Similarly, a flexible cane or 'lathi' may be used in some countries, such as India, to compress and lift the larynx.

There may be scratches and bruises on the neck, which may have been caused when the victim tried to pull off the ligature, or when there had also been attempts at manual strangulation preceding or following the application of a ligature.

Internally, similar findings to those seen in manual strangulation may be found, but damage is usually less and areas of bruising less localized. Fractures of the larynx are less common and the haemorrhage in the neck muscle is often more localized.

Ligature strangulation is best treated as homicide until it is shown conclusively not to be so. Accidents do happen in which ligatures pass around the neck and become tightened and it is certainly possible for a person to kill themselves by ligature strangulation, although this is most uncommon.

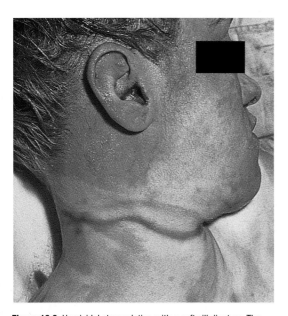

Figure 13.6 Homicidal strangulation with a soft silk ligature. The folding of the material has caused the deep grooved mark and the fainter red mark above it.

HANGING

Hanging or 'self-suspension' is a form of ligature strangulation in which the pressure of the ligature on the neck is produced by the weight of the body itself. Hanging need not be from a high point of suspension with the body hanging fully free under gravity and with the feet clear of the ground, although this is what often happens. Many hanging deaths occur in which the victim is slumped in a sitting, kneeling or half-lying position, being suspended from a low point such as a door handle, bed knob etc.

Most hangings, especially the free-swinging positions, show none of the 'classical signs' of asphyxia, as death has occurred almost instantaneously, presumably from sudden pressure on the neck producing vagal inhibition. Low-point hangings, on the other hand, may show florid asphyxial changes, which indicate that death is not due to vagal inhibition.

LIVERPOOL JOHN MOORES UNIVERSITY
LEARNING SERVICES

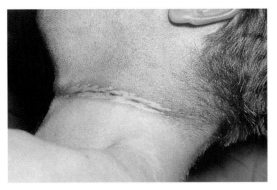

Figure 13.7 The spiral weave of the rope can be seen in this horizontal ligature mark caused by hanging from a low suspension point. The appearances may mimic homicidal ligature strangulation.

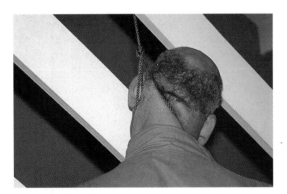

Figure 13.8 Suicidal hanging: the rope rises to a point, leaving a gap in the ligature mark – the suspension point – on the neck.

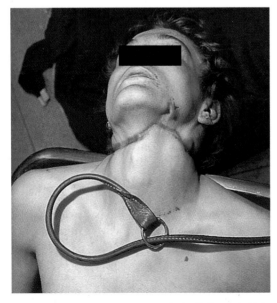

Figure 13.9 Suicidal hanging with a dog lead, with the mark rising to a suspension point at the front of the neck.

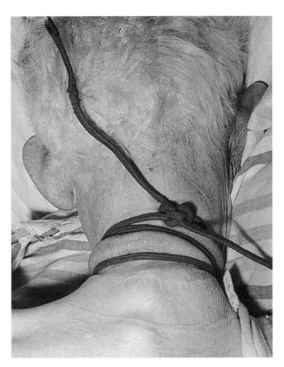

Figure 13.10 Suicidal strangulation with a cable. The initial appearances were those of homicide, but a full examination of the circumstances indicated suicide.

The cause of death in the hanging for judicial execution is quite different, as the arrested drop of several metres completely disrupts the cervical spine, sometimes at the atlanto-occipital joint, but usually in the mid-cervical portion. No asphyxial signs are seen in properly performed judicial hangings. It is very unusual for the cervical spine to be broken in suicidal hanging unless there has been an unusually long drop.

The usual free-swinging suicidal hanging shows a mark on the neck that is somewhat sloped and does not run around the full circumference of the neck. The junction of the noose and the vertical part of the rope of the noose is pulled upwards and away from the skin and so no mark is left. The apex of the triangle formed in this way is called the suspension 'peak' or 'point' and indicates the position of the junction of the noose and vertical part of rope. This suspension peak or point is a distinguishing feature from ligature strangulation.

Excluding judicial execution, hanging is mostly commonly a suicidal act of males. Some cases are accidental and entanglement with cords and ropes can occur; amongst children, many tragedies have happened due to leather or plastic restraint harnesses getting around the necks of unattended infants. The tying

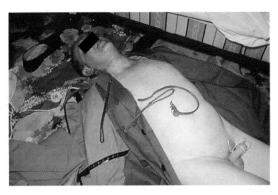

Figure 13.11 Sexual asphyxia by a dog collar and lead. The lead had been attached to the ankles so that pressure could be applied to the neck.

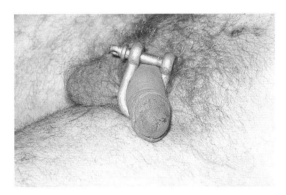

Figure 13.12 Sexual asphyxia is commonly associated with other paraphilias.

of toys to the sides of cots results in several deaths of young children each year. ·

THE SEXUAL ASPHYXIAS

The most common accidental hangings occur in the sexual asphyxias and it is important for doctors to be aware of this situation, as many have been mislabelled suicide or even homicide by the investigative authorities. These acts are almost totally confined to men, usually between puberty and middle age; they are almost unknown in women. Essentially, it is believed by some that cerebral hypoxia, commonly achieved by some form of pressure on the neck, increases the sexual experience. The aim of the individual, therefore, is to achieve sufficient hypoxia for his own needs and, once the sexual gratification is obtained, to release the mechanism(s) used to achieve the hypoxia

and return to normality. Occasionally, the device malfunctions or the design is not 'fail safe' and death ensues. It is very common for the noose to be padded, so that no bruising to the neck will be caused. Hypoxia may also be induced by masks, pads on the face or envelopment in plastic. The scene will often show signs of sexual activity, with pornography within sight of the victim, and all permutations of unusual and bizarre clothing, props and behaviour may be seen in association with these deaths, but in most cases they must be regarded as accidents.

TRAUMATIC ASPHYXIA

The essential feature is fixation of the thorax by external pressure that prevents respiratory movements. This is perhaps one of the purest types of asphyxia and it is the one in which the classic signs of congestion, cyanosis and petechiae are often seen in their most gross form. There is commonly florid red or blue congestion of the face and neck, which usually ceases at the level of the clavicles. The eyes may show extensive petechiae and ecchymoses; the bleeding may even be so gross as to form blood blisters protruding through the eyelids from the haemorrhagic conjunctivae. For some reason, which is not fully understood, immobilization of respiratory movements causes a very marked rise in venous pressure in the head and neck, which is perhaps due to the failure of chest expansion to aid the return of blood to the right side of the heart. The victim may also show injuries from the compressing agent but, if the pressure has been broad, there may be no mark of trauma on the body.

'Postural asphyxia' is a related condition, in which an unconscious or disabled person lies with the upper half of the body lower than the remainder; the common example is the drunk who slides out of bed so that his head is on the floor. This inverted position means that the abdominal viscera push up against and splint the diaphragm and this can cause death. This is generally a slow process and, as a result, there is usually marked cyanosis, congestion and petechiae in the face and neck. If the body is not found quickly, some of these changes may be made to appear worse by postmortem hypostasis in the dependent areas.

Deaths with an aetiology somewhere between traumatic and postural asphyxia have occurred during restraint when several policemen or prison officers have forced prisoners to the ground and then knelt on

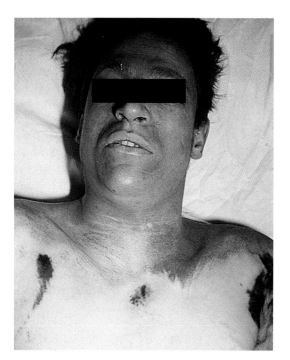

Figure 13.13 Traumatic asphyxia due to pressure on the chest from an overturned tractor. The extensive congestion and petechial haemorrhages in the head and neck are typical of this type of asphyxia.

or otherwise pressed on their thorax. The difficulty of having to raise some of their own body weight with their respiratory muscles to breathe, combined with the additional pressure of others pressing on their chest, may cause these individuals to be unable to breathe sufficiently frequently or deeply and they will gradually asphyxiate. Unusually for a death due to traumatic or postural asphyxia, the congestion, cyanosis and petechial haemorrhages are minimal or absent, suggesting a different mode of death.

It is now well accepted that if any individual, especially after violent struggle, is handcuffed and forced on to the ground face down or placed into a police vehicle face down, his respiratory movements will become difficult or impossible to maintain against the weight of his own body and asphyxia may ensue. These individuals should be placed on their side or, better still, sat upright. Kneeling on the chest or any other form of chest compression during restraint is now accepted as being potentially fatal, and both the police and the prison service in the UK teach their officers of the risks of such pressure.

Chapter fourteen

Immersion and Drowning

Signs of immersion   Drowning   Laboratory tests for drowning

Bodies recovered from water may have:

- died of natural causes before entering the water;
- died of natural causes while in the water, having entered the water either voluntarily or accidentally;
- died from exposure and hypothermia in the water;
- died of injuries or other unnatural cause before entering the water;
- died of injuries after entering the water;
- died from submersion, but not drowning; or
- died from true drowning as a result of aspiration of water into the lungs.

SIGNS OF IMMERSION

It is essential to appreciate that the signs of immersion are unrelated to drowning. Any dead body, whatever the cause of death, will develop signs of immersion if left for a sufficient time in water.

The earliest stages of immersion are commonly seen in those who spend a long time with their hands immersed in water: the skin of the tips of the fingers becomes somewhat opaque and wrinkled. These changes, known as 'washerwoman's fingers', develop after a few hours in cold water (and a shorter time in warm water) as the skin, but especially the thick keratin layers on the palms and soles, becomes macerated and appears white and wrinkled. After a few days, this macerated skin will begin to separate and, usually

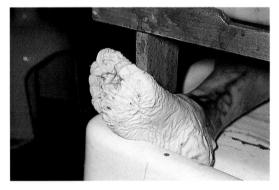

Figure 14.1 'Washerwoman' changes in the foot of a body that had been in water for several weeks.

within 1–2 weeks (again depending on temperature), the skin will peel off the hands and feet.

It is often claimed that another early sign of immersion is cutis anserina or 'gooseflesh', which is a widespread pimpling of the skin due to contraction of the errector pili muscles. However, this is partly due to cold (and may be seen in refrigerated bodies) and partly due to rigor mortis; it is not seen in the bathtub users. Cutis anserina is not a specific sign of immersion.

Most of the other signs of immersion are due to the decomposition of the body. As a very rough guide, in average temperate conditions a body immersed in water will decompose at about half the speed of one left in air. After about a week, the body will be bloated and the face, abdomen and genitals will be distended with

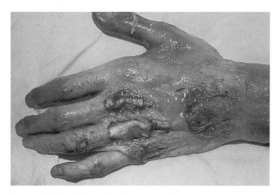

Figure 14.2 Hand from a body recovered from a shallow river showing the effects of post-mortem trauma against the river bed.

gas. After about 2 weeks' immersion in temperate conditions, the skin and hair become loose and will begin to detach. Bodies immersed in water are often not discovered until they float to the surface and the time at which this happens is very variable and is dependent on the extent of gas accumulation and also on the body weight. Obese people and some women may sink for only a short period due to the effect of fat.

Post-mortem artefactual damage, including the effects of predators – fish, crustaceans, molluscs and reptiles, rodents, dogs and, in some countries, larger animals – will increase the rate of decomposition. As the body decomposes, so the tissues will become increasingly fragile and will fragment and detach easily until, eventually, skeletalization occurs.

As the body is moved by the flow of the water, contact with rocks, piers and many other underwater obstructions can cause damage. These post-mortem injuries must be differentiated from ante-mortem injuries that may be evidence of criminal violence. Certain injuries are unique to bodies immersed in water, for instance the parallel sliced lacerations characteristic of a rapidly revolving propeller of a motorboat.

DROWNING

The mechanism of death in true drowning is not one of simple hypoxia from deprivation of air. The exact effects on the body and the abnormalities that are caused by the entry of water into the airways differ according to the type of water in which drowning occurs: hypotonic or hypertonic.

Fresh water is hypotonic compared to plasma, so that when water enters the lungs, a rapid transfer of fluid takes place from the alveoli into the vascular system through the alveolar membranes because of the osmotic difference between the water in the lungs and the plasma. This transfer of fluids may increase the blood volume by as much as 50 per cent within a minute and this hypervolaemia will place a great strain on the heart. The rapid influx of water will render the plasma hypotonic, which in turn will result in haemolysis of red blood cells, and major shifts in the plasma electrolytes will occur extremely rapidly. It was once thought that severe hyperkalaemia caused by the release of potassium from the haemolysed red blood cells contributed significantly to rapid myocardial failure, but more recent work has shown this to be only a relatively minor factor in death in fresh-water drowning.

Seawater is hypertonic, so that water is withdrawn by osmosis from the plasma into the fluid in the alveolar spaces in the lungs. There is also electrolyte transfer, with mainly sodium and chloride passing from the hypertonic inhaled fluid into the blood. The lack of hypervolaemia, with the consequent absence of strain on the heart, probably accounts for the longer survival times in salt-water submersion.

In all types of drowning, the deprivation of oxygen caused by obstruction of the alveolar spaces is, of course, a factor, especially as the time of immersion lengthens. As in all kinds of hypoxia, irreversible cortical brain damage will occur if oxygenated blood fails to perfuse the brain for more than a number of minutes. It was formerly thought that 3 minutes was the threshold of danger and this may still be so in many cases, but oxygen deprivation times of over 10 minutes with complete recovery of brain function have been recorded, although these are likely to be the rare exception rather than the rule. Where hypothermia also exists, particularly when it has a rapid onset, such as in immersion in very cold water or immersion of a child, the total immersion time compatible with full brain recovery can be far longer and can even, on very rare occasions, be in excess of 40 minutes.

The post-mortem findings in either type of drowning, whether on external observation or at autopsy, may be variable. Drowning is one of the most difficult modes of death to prove at post mortem, especially when the body is not examined in a fresh condition. Classically, there will be a plume of froth at the mouth and nostrils, which may sometimes be tinged with blood. This froth fills the air passages and exudes on to the face. It is composed of water containing plasma protein and surfactant that has been whipped into a froth by the violent terminal respiratory actions. The plume of froth is more common in drowning in hypertonic seawater. Externally this may be the only sign, but it is absent more often than it is present, especially when the body has been dead for some time.

Internally, froth may still be found in the trachea and bronchi for some time after death, but eventually even this vanishes as decomposition begins. When the sternum is removed at autopsy, the lungs may be seen to be over-distended, filling the thorax and covering the anterior surface of the heart, which is normally exposed. The lungs may have a 'doughy' texture and remain inflated and spongy to the touch. There may be blurred areas of haemolysed blood under the pleura, but only rarely are there any true petechiae.

Dissection of the lung may show generalized pulmonary oedema, but where any water in the air spaces has been absorbed into the pulmonary circulation, the oedema will be absent – this is the so-called 'dry-lung drowning'.

The mechanism of death in individuals who die as a result of submersion is not always classical drowning. In a significant proportion of cases, the person dies quickly, sometimes within seconds of entering the water. The mode of death of these cases is considered to be cardiac arrest, which is most likely to be due to a vagal inhibitory reflex triggered by a sudden stimulation of sensitive areas. It is known that falling into cold water can initiate this reflex, either by rapid cooling of the body surface or by a sudden inrush of cold water into the mouth and nasal passages impinging on the sensitive mucosa of the pharynx and larynx.

Sudden death on entering water is more likely in drunken people, in whom the skin is flushed from alcohol-induced vasodilatation, and sailors falling into a harbour on their way back from heavy drinking in the local bars are a common example of this type of death. This type of very rapid death on immersion is also said to occur in emotionally tense individuals (such as intending suicides), in whom the nervous reflex arcs seem more active.

LABORATORY TESTS FOR DROWNING

The diatom test depends on the presence of microscopic algae, called diatoms, which are often, but not always, present in seawater and unpolluted natural fresh water. There are about 25 000 species of diatom and all have an almost indestructible silicaceous capsule. The theory behind the test is that normal people do not have significant numbers of diatoms in the kidneys, brain, marrow etc., but if a person drowns in diatom-containing water, the algae in that water will reach the lungs and some of them will penetrate the alveolar walls. If the heart is still beating, the diatoms that have entered the bloodstream will be transported around the body in the circulation and may lodge in distant organs such as the kidney, brain and bone marrow before death. An increase in the number of diatoms in the internal organs was thought to confirm that the body had drowned and, if a sample of the

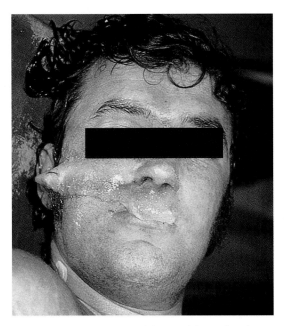

Figure 14.3 Profuse blood-tinged froth around the mouth and nose in drowning.

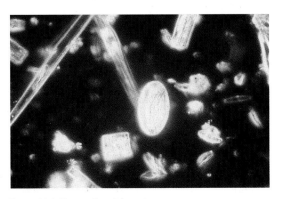

Figure 14.4 Diatoms from lake water.

water was also taken at the presumed site of drowning, the similarity of different species of diatom in the water and the body could be compared.

On the other hand, if a dead body was dropped into water, although diatoms could reach the lung by passive percolation, no circulatory transfer could occur and so (theoretically) no diatoms would be present in the distant organs. The advantages claimed for this technique include the fact that it could be used even in the presence of putrefaction, if protected tissue such as bone marrow was examined.

Unfortunately, the diatom test is often negative, even in undoubted cases of drowning in waterways full of diatoms, and there have been numerous false-positive results that are said to have occurred for a variety of technical reasons. All in all, this test is now so unreliable that it should only be used, and the results interpreted, with great circumspection.

Many attempts have been made to identify a chemical test or some other type of analysis of the blood that will assist in the diagnosis of either fresh-water or seawater drowning. Analyses of the concentrations of sodium, chloride and magnesium have been used, but the results are too variable (due to the rapid post-mortem diffusion of electrolytes throughout the body after death) to be of any practical use.

Chapter fifteen

Injury due to Heat, Cold and Electricity

Heat, cold and electricity are some of the 'physical agents' that can cause non-kinetic injuries to the body.

INJURY DUE TO HEAT

Exposure of living tissue to high temperatures will cause damage to the cells. The extent of the damage caused is a function of the length of time of exposure as well as of the temperature to which the tissues are exposed. Damage to the skin can occur at temperatures as low as 44°C if exposed for several hours; at temperatures over 50°C or so, damage occurs more rapidly, and at 60°C tissue damage occurs in 3 seconds.

The heat source may be dry or wet; where the heat is dry, the resultant injury is called a 'burn', whereas with moist heat from hot water, steam and other hot liquids it is known as 'scalding'.

Burning

Dry burns are classified by both severity and extent. There are several systems of classification of the severity of burns, the most useful of which is:

1 first degree – erythema and blistering (vesiculation);
2 second degree – burning of the whole thickness of the epidermis and exposure of the dermis;
3 third degree – destruction down to subdermal tissues, sometimes with carbonization and exposure of muscle and bone.

The size of the area of the burning may be more important in the assessment of the dangers of the burn than the depth. The 'Rule of Nines' is used to calculate the approximate extent on the body surface. Where the burnt area exceeds 50 per cent, the prognosis is poor, even in first-degree burns. The age of the individual is also important: the elderly may die with only 20 per cent burns, whereas children and young adults are generally more resilient. There is, of course, considerable individual variation and the speed and extent of emergency treatment will play a significant part in the morbidity and mortality of burns' victims. In dry burns, any clothing will offer some protection against heat unless it ignites.

Scalds

The general features of scalds are similar to those of burns, with erythema and blistering, but charring of the skin is only found when the liquid is extremely hot, such as with molten metal. The pattern of scalding will depend upon the way in which the body has been exposed to the fluid: immersion into hot liquid results in an upper 'fluid level', whereas splashed or

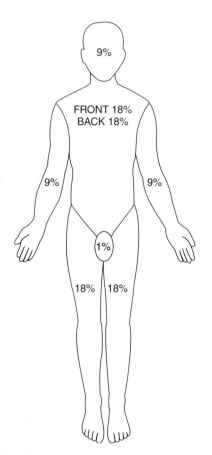

Figure 15.1 The 'Rule of Nines'.

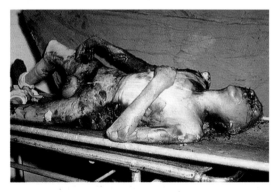

Figure 15.2 Burns in a victim of a house fire.

scattered droplets of liquid result in scattered punctate areas of scalding. Runs or dribbles of hot fluid will leave characteristic areas of scalding – these runs or dribbles will generally flow under the influence of gravity and this can provide a marker to the orientation of the victim at the time the fluid was moving.

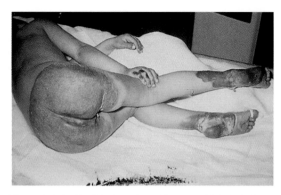

Figure 15.3 Scalds of the buttocks and feet on a child who had been dipped into a bath of extremely hot water as a punishment.

If only small quantities of liquid hit the skin, cooling will be rapid, which will reduce the amount of damage done to the skin. However, if clothing is soaked by hot fluid, the underlying skin may be badly affected, as the fabric will retain the hot liquid against the skin surface. Scalding is seen in industrial accidents where steam pipes or boilers burst and it is also seen in children who pull kettles and cooking pots down upon themselves. Scalds are also seen in child physical abuse when a child is placed in a tub or bath of hot water.

The examination of bodies recovered from fires

Not all bodies recovered from fires have burnt to death; in fact, the majority of deaths in fires are the result of inhalation of smoke and noxious gases (cyanide, carbon monoxide, oxides of nitrogen, phosgene etc.). Bodies recovered from the scene of a fire may have been burnt both before and after death and it can be difficult or impossible to differentiate these burns, especially where considerable destruction has taken place. As a general guide, the ante-mortem burn usually has broad, erythematous margins with blisters both in the burned area and along the edge, whereas post-mortem burns tend to lack this erythema or it is at least less pronounced. It is now accepted that heat applied to the recently dead body (certainly up to at least 60 minutes after cardiac arrest) can still produce a red flare of erythema, and so great care must be taken in any attempt to determine the time at which a burn was caused.

Blisters are produced as a result of the heat trauma and can be either ante mortem or post mortem. It has

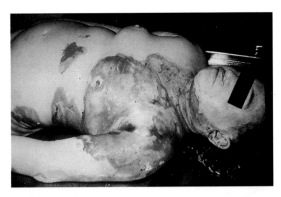

Figure 15.4 A mixture of ante-mortem and post-mortem burns from ignited clothing. Differentiating peri-mortem burns is extremely difficult.

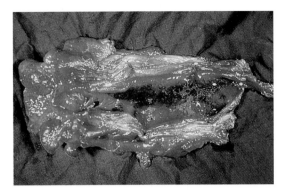

Figure 15.6 Trachea showing soot and mucus following inhalation of fire fumes and smoke.

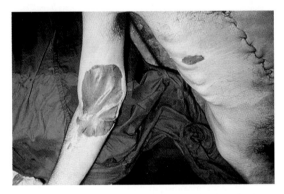

Figure 15.5 Post-mortem burns of the arm and the chest due to a hot-water bottle used in an attempt at resuscitation being left in contact with the body.

been claimed that ante-mortem blisters contain a fluid with a high protein content, whereas post-mortem vesicles have a more aqueous fluid; this is rarely a practical means of differentiation, even if true.

Fire is a good means of attempting to conceal (or at least confuse) the injuries and other marks that may indicate that the deceased was a victim of homicide. It will almost certainly cause some destruction of forensically useful evidence. As a result, all burnt bodies must be viewed with particular care and the possibility that the death might have occurred before the fire began must be considered. The scene should be examined by specialist fire investigators, with the assistance of the pathologist if necessary. The position of the body when discovered is important because sometimes, when flames or smoke are advancing, the victim will retreat into a corner, a cupboard or other hiding place, or they may simply move to a place furthest away from the fire or to a doorway or window, all of

which may indicate that the victim was probably still alive and capable of movement for some time after the start of the fire.

The colour of the skin in areas that have been protected from burns and smoke staining should be noted; if they are 'cherry-pink', this indicates that the blood is very likely to contain significant quantities of carboxyhaemoglobin. Similar pink appearances can be seen on internal examination, particularly of the brain and the skeletal muscles. These appearances must be confirmed by toxicological analysis. Other features that indicate that the victim was alive and breathing while the fire was burning are the presence of soot particles in the larynx, trachea and bronchi, where they are commonly associated with mucus, and evidence of heat trauma to the mucosa. Soot in the nostrils and perhaps mouth should be assumed to have entered passively.

The findings of soot in the airways and carbon monoxide in the blood indicate that the person was breathing after the fire began. However, it must be strongly emphasized that the converse is not true: the absence of soot and carbon monoxide certainly does not mean that the victim must have been dead before the fire started. The absence of these signs is more common in rapid flash fires, such as gasoline (petrol) conflagrations in cars or light aircraft, where little soot or carbon monoxide is produced.

Causes of death in burns and scalds

The actual cause of death from burns is complex and results from the interplay of many factors. In rapid deaths, the directly destructive effects of heat on the respiratory tract leading to asphyxia, the combined toxic effects of carbon monoxide, cyanide and the multitude of other noxious gases (oxides of nitrogen, phosgene etc.) that are inhaled, the release of toxic material from the extensive tissue destruction, and 'shock' due to pain all cause or contribute to death. Most of these factors do not apply to scalds, unless the victim falls into the hot liquid.

Where death from burns or scalds is delayed, dehydration and electrolyte disturbances as a result of plasma loss from the damaged skin surfaces are early causes of death. Later, renal failure, toxaemia from substances absorbed from the burned area and infection of widespread burns may be responsible (see Chapter 16).

Injuries on burned bodies

A careful search must be made for any ante-mortem injuries that may have caused or contributed to death. These injuries can be of almost any type, but strangulation and shooting appear to be most common in cases of homicide concealed by fire. It is always advisable to x-ray a burned body, especially if the fire damage is so extensive as to make examination of the skin surface impossible.

However, not all injuries on burned bodies are sinister, and where skin has been subjected to severe burning or charring, it will often split. These splits can also be caused by post-mortem movement during recovery of the body when charred and brittle skin is moved. These injuries sometimes worry the police or fire brigade, who suspect that they are due to previous injury, but their appearance, position and lack of any ante-mortem tissue response are usually a clear indication of their post-mortem nature.

Another misinterpreted injury is the 'heat haematoma' inside the skull. This spurious 'extradural haematoma' lies between the bone and dura and is caused when severe heat has been applied to the scalp, resulting in expansion of the blood in the skull diplöe and the intracranial venous sinuses, which rupture, resulting in the formation of a collection of blood outside the meninges. The blood is brown and spongy, unlike a true haematoma, but the simple presence of this collection of blood may mislead the unwary doctor performing an autopsy into thinking that this is the result of a trauma.

There is seldom any doubt about the cause of these collections of blood. However, it has been said that if

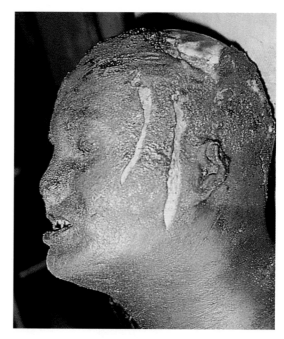

Figure 15.7 Skin splits in the victim of a house fire. These splits were initially thought to be incised wounds.

there is carboxyhaemoglobin in the peripheral blood, then if the haematoma is due to heat, it will also contain carboxyhaemoglobin. On the other hand, a true extradural haematoma, which had developed before the fire began, will not contain any appreciable amount of carboxyhaemoglobin. The test is not fool proof, but may be a useful adjunct to other methods of investigation.

COLD INJURY (HYPOTHERMIA)

Hypothermia has both clinical and forensic aspects, as many people suffer from and die of hypothermia even in temperate climates in winter. In marine disasters, hypothermia may be as common a cause of death as drowning. In the very cold waters of seas and lakes in high latitudes, death from immersion may occur within a couple of minutes from sheer heat loss and before true drowning can occur.

In practice, most deaths from hypothermia are seen in old people and in some children, both of whom are particularly vulnerable to hypothermia. Old people may become severely hypothermic due to their restricted economic circumstances or to senile mental changes, and for a number of reasons they may go without adequate heating, food and clothing. An added factor may be myxoedema, which predisposes to low body temperature, or the use of phenothiazine drugs, which also predisposes towards hypothermia. It is important to remember that the weather does not have to be unusually cold for hypothermia to develop and, even in moderately cold winter weather, many elderly individuals will become hypothermic.

Children have a high body surface-to-weight ratio and lose heat rapidly. In some cases of deliberate neglect or careless family circumstances, infants may be left in unheated rooms in winter and suffer hypothermia. Another group includes drunken people, who may collapse or lie down to sleep after too much alcohol and become hypothermic, especially because alcohol causes vasodilatation of the skin, increasing heat loss.

The signs of hypothermia

Any fall in body core temperature of more than a few degrees is hypothermia, but clinical effects are slight providing the core body temperature remains above about 35°C. The body has a series of mechanisms to raise the body temperature, including diversion of blood away from the skin and shivering. Below 32°C, shivering ceases and thus this extra muscular activity will no longer generate heat, and so the situation worsens. People whose temperature falls to 28°C or less are almost certain to die, even with treatment.

When a dead person is found and hypothermia is suspected, it can be difficult or impossible to prove because post-mortem cooling (including storage in a mortuary refrigerator) can cause some similar changes to appear in the skin. However, if the body shows areas with indistinct, blurred margins that are pink or brown-pink, particularly over and around joints such as the knees, elbows and hips and also in sites where they cannot be due to hypostasis due to their distribution, a diagnosis of hypothermia should be considered. The pink colour is due to unreduced oxyhaemoglobin as the cold tissues have little uptake of oxygen. The cause of the rather blurred, brownish tinge around the joints is unclear, but suggests that there may be a degree of red cell haemolysis. Very rarely, hypothermic victims will have blisters in the affected areas of skin.

Internally, there may be no signs at all, but quite commonly, the stomach lining is studded with numerous brown-black acute erosions, which are exactly the

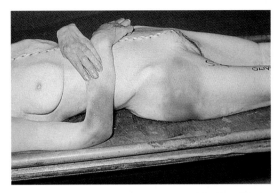

Figure 15.8 Discoloration of the skin in a case of fatal hypothermia.

same as those seen in many types of pre-death stress. Increased viscosity of the blood due to low temperatures may lead to sludging of blood in the small vessels of many organs and this may lead to micro-infarcts. This mechanism is probably the cause of the haemorrhagic pancreatitis and associated fat necrosis that are also features of many cases of hypothermia.

Hypothermia may be linked with a strange condition, particularly in the elderly, in which people take off some or all of their clothing (reciprocal undressing). They may then hide themselves in corners, in cupboards or under piles of furniture or household goods. This is called the 'hide-and-die syndrome' and is well known. An alternative, and perhaps more common, scenario is of a naked or partly clothed elderly individual found amid a scene of utter confusion with furniture pulled over and drawers and cupboards emptied out. Close examination of the scene will show that all of the disturbance is at low level and that the tops of tables etc. are not disturbed. When bodies are found in either of these situations, the police may be suspicious of some criminal action, but examination of the scene and the post-mortem features of hypothermia will explain these worrying circumstances.

If hypothermia of the extremities has been present for a long time, there may be 'frost-bite', which is infarction of the peripheral digits with oedema, redness and later necrosis of the tissue beyond a line of inflammatory demarcation. There need not be any generalized associated hypothermia.

ELECTRICAL INJURY

Injury and death from the passage of an electric current through the body are common in both industrial and domestic circumstances. The essential factor in causing harm is the current (i.e. an electron flow) which is measured in milliamperes (mA). This in turn is determined by the resistance of the tissues in ohms and the voltage of the power supply in volts (V), according to Ohm's Law. To increase the current (and hence the damage), either the resistance must fall or the voltage must increase, or both.

Almost all cases of electrocution, fatal or otherwise, originate from the public power supply, which is delivered throughout the world at either 110 or 240 V. It is rare for death to occur at less than 100 V. The current needed to produce death varies according to the time during which it passes and the part of the body across which it flows. Usually, the entry point is a hand that touches an electrical appliance or live conductor, and the exit is to earth (or 'ground'), often via the other hand or the feet. In either case, the current will cross the thorax, the most dangerous area for a shock because of the risks of cardiac arrest or respiratory paralysis.

When a live metal conductor is gripped by the hand, pain and muscle twitching will occur if the current reaches about 10 mA. If the current in the arm exceeds about 30 mA, the muscles will go into spasm, which cannot be voluntarily released because the flexor muscles are stronger than the extensors; the result is for the hand to grip or to 'hold on'. This 'hold-on' effect is very dangerous as it may allow the circuit to be maintained for long enough to cause cardiac arrhythmia, whereas the normal response would have been to let go so as to stop the pain.

If the current across the chest is 50 mA or more, even for only a few seconds, fatal ventricular fibrillation is likely to occur, and alternating current (AC – very common in domestic supplies) is much more dangerous than direct current (DC) at precipitating cardiac arrhythmias.

The tissue resistance is important. Thick dry skin, such as the palm of the hand or sole of the foot, may have a resistance of 1 million ohms (Ω), but when wet, this may fall to a few hundred ohms and the current, given a fixed supply voltage, will be markedly increased. This is relevant in wet conditions such as bathrooms, exterior building sites or when sweating.

The mode of death in most cases of electrocution is ventricular fibrillation due to the direct effects of the current on the myocardium and cardiac conducting system. These changes can be reversed when the current ceases, which may explain some of the remarkable recoveries following prolonged cardiac massage after receipt of an electric shock. The victims of such an arrhythmia will be pale, whereas those who die as a result of peripheral respiratory paralysis are usually cyanosed. Even more rare are the instances in which the current has entered the head and caused primary brainstem paralysis, which has resulted in failure of respiration. This may occur when workers on overhead power supply lines or electric railway wires touch their heads against high-tension conductors, usually 660 V.

The electrical lesion

Unless the circumstances are accurately known, it can be difficult to know whether a dead victim has been in contact with electricity. When high voltages or prolonged contact have occurred, extensive and severe burns can be seen, but a few seconds' contact with a faulty appliance may leave minimal signs. Where the skin is wet or where the body is immersed, as in a bath, there may be no signs at all, as the entrance and exit of the current may be spread over such a wide area that no focal lesion exists.

Usually, however, there is a discrete focal point of entry and, as the electrical current is concentrated at that point, enough energy can be released to cause a thermal lesion. The entry points may be multiple and obvious, or they may be single and very inconspicuous. As the most commonplace is on the hands, these should always be examined with particular care.

The focal electrical lesion is usually a blister, which occurs when the conductor is in firm contact with the skin and which usually collapses soon after infliction, forming a raised rim with a concave centre. The skin is pale, often white, and an areola of pallor (due to local vasoconstriction) is a characteristic feature. The blister may vary from a few millimetres to several centimetres. The skin often peels off the large blisters leaving a red base. The other type of electrical mark is a 'spark burn', where there is an air gap between metal and skin. Here, a central nodule of fused keratin, brown or yellow in colour, is surrounded by the typical areola of pale skin. Both types of lesion often lie adjacent to each other. In high-voltage burns, multiple sparks may crackle onto the victim and cause large areas of damage, sometimes called 'crocodile skin' due to its appearance.

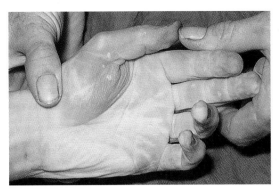

Figure 15.9 Multiple minute electrical marks on the hand caused by contact with a faulty electrical drill.

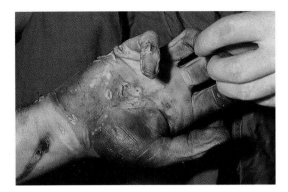

Figure 15.12 Extensive electrical burns with scorching and blistering.

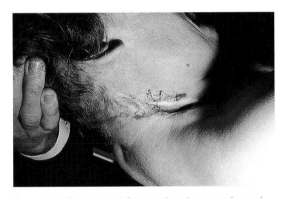

Figure 15.10 Electrical mark from a mains wire wrapped around the neck. There is marked hyperaemia and adjacent pallor, with evidence of blistering.

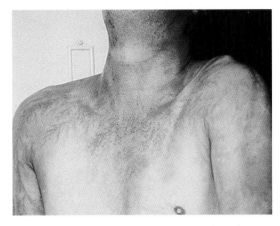

Figure 15.13 The fern-like pattern of a lightning strike can be seen on the upper chest.

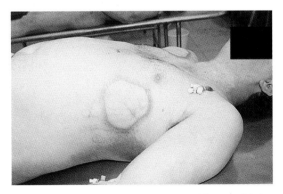

Figure 15.11 Hyperaemia from a defibrillator paddle, caused during attempted resuscitation.

Internally, there are no characteristic findings in fatal electrocution. The skin lesions are mainly thermal in nature, but opinions vary as to whether histological appearances are specific to electricity. It has been said that the cell nuclei line up in parallel rows due to the electric field, but similar appearances can occur in purely thermal burns. There are specific intracellular lesions on electron microscopy, but the gross pathological diagnosis relies upon the external appearances.

DEATH FROM LIGHTNING

Hundreds of deaths occur each year from atmospheric lightning, especially in tropical countries. A lightning strike from cloud to earth may involve property, animals or humans. Huge electrical forces are involved, producing millions of amperes and phenomenal voltages. Some of the lesions caused to those who are struck directly or simply caught close to the lightning strike are electrical, but other will be from burns and yet others are due to the compression wave of heated air, which is like an explosion. All kinds of bizarre appearances may be found, especially the partial or complete stripping of clothing from the victim, which may arouse suspicions of foul play. Severe burns, fractures and gross lacerations can occur, along with the well-known magnetization or even fusion of metallic objects in the clothing. The usual textbook description is of 'fern or branch-like' patterns on the skin, but in fact most bodies do not show this. Red streaks following skin creases or sweat-damped tracks are more likely, though many bodies are completely unmarked.

Chapter sixteen

Effects of Injuries

Haemorrhage	Pulmonary thrombo-embolism	**Adult respiratory distress syndrome**
Infection	Foreign-body embolism	**Suprarenal haemorrhage**
Embolism	Amniotic fluid embolism	**Subendocardial haemorrhages**
Fat embolism	**Disseminated intravascular**	
Air embolism	**coagulation**	

Some injuries are so severe that they are immediately and obviously incompatible with life, for instance the gross disruption of a body caused by an explosion. Minimal injuries, for example abrasions, are extremely unlikely to lead to any significant degree of incapacity, let alone disability or death. Between these two ends of the spectrum lie a wide range of types and severity of injuries that may or may not result in incapacity, disability or death. The effects of trauma depend not only on the severity of the injury but also on the response of the individual to that particular trauma.

The forensic practitioner must understand both the immediate and the long-term effects of trauma in order to be able to explain those effects to a court or to the relatives.

HAEMORRHAGE

External bleeding is usually obvious; internal bleeding is very commonly confined to the body cavities, tissue spaces or directly into large organs such as the lungs or the liver. Bleeding within the skull is dangerous because of the space-occupying effect of the collection of blood upon the brain, and the same may be said about bleeding into the pericardial sac and its effect on the heart.

The speed of blood loss is crucial. An adult human can rapidly lose approximately 10 per cent of their total blood volume without there being a significant effect on the stability of their cardiovascular system. The effects of blood loss are rapidly compensated by a powerful sympathetic response, which constricts both the arterioles and the great veins and results in an increase in the heart rate, which has the effect of maintaining blood pressure and circulating blood volume. Endocrine responses including vasopressin and angiotensin also play their part in the longer term. This is described as non-progressive or compensated shock.

If more blood is lost, the protective reflexes are overwhelmed: the blood pressure will begin to fall, which will have adverse effects upon the heart and, as the myocardium begins to deteriorate, there is a further fall of blood pressure and a worsening of the vicious cycle. Other effects of the falling blood pressure include failure of the sympathetic centres themselves, thrombosis, increased capillary permeability and the release of toxins from damaged or dead tissues. This is called progressive shock and will result in death if treatment is not given.

If bleeding continues, a third stage of shock is reached during which treatment may have a temporarily beneficial effect but will not affect the ultimately fatal outcome. This is called irreversible shock. The time scale for these various stages of shock is very variable and depends, among other things, upon the rate of blood loss and the previous health of the individual.

The forensic practitioner is often asked how much activity the injured individual would have been capable of performing and for how long. These questions can only be answered in the broadest terms: some victims will be rapidly incapacitated, whereas others, with equally severe injuries, may be able to continue to run, fight or operate controls for a considerable time.

Any opinion about the amount of blood found at a scene must be made with caution: small amounts of blood can sometimes cover very large areas, whereas large amounts of blood lost onto absorbent surfaces such as carpets may not appear significant. Remember that wounds can continue to bleed after death, sometimes copiously, due to passive leakage.

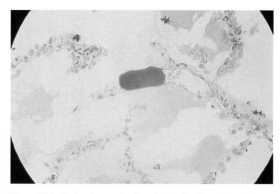

Figure 16.1 Photomicrograph of lung stained with osmic acid to show the globule of fat in the alveolar capillary following a fractured tibia.

INFECTION

Prompt treatment by adequate modern medical services will almost completely eliminate the risk of significant infection following wounding. However, without adequate treatment, even minor wounds can cause death from infection. Many types of organism can be involved, the most common being staphylococci, streptococci, coliforms, *Pseudomonas aeruginosa* and the anaerobes such as *Clostridium perfringens* and *C. tetani*. Localized infection may develop into frank septicaemia and 'septic shock', which has a high mortality.

EMBOLISM

An embolus is a solid, liquid or gas that is not normally found in the blood and that is carried in the blood flow through the vascular system until it can travel no further because it has become lodged in a small blood vessel or across the bifurcation of a larger vessel. The exact behaviour and effect of an embolus depend upon its physical characteristics and its site.

Fat embolism

Fat embolism is associated with fractures of the long bones and trauma to areas rich in adipose tissue. Microscopic examination of sections of lung specifically stained for fat will commonly show a few fat globules after almost any tissue trauma, and even normal lungs may reveal a few fat deposits. Pulmonary fat embolism may therefore have no clinical consequences unless it is so gross as to cause hypoxia by widespread obstruction of capillaries. The pulmonary capillaries can only retain a certain amount of fat and, if that threshold is exceeded, the fat will appear in the systemic circulation. This may possibly account for the usual delay of hours or even a day or so between injury and death from fat embolism. Others suggest that the source of the fat in the bloodstream is not from the injured tissue but rather from changes in fat metabolism and transport as a result of the trauma.

Free fat in the systemic circulation can have much more serious effects, and fat emboli may be found microscopically in many organs including the brain, kidneys and myocardium. Systemic fat emboli in the skin and retina are often associated with small areas of haemorrhage, which can be seen, both in the living and in those who subsequently die, as petechiae. Obstruction of the arterioles causes micro-infarcts in many organs, which, if they involve the brainstem or the myocardium, can be rapidly fatal.

Fat embolism may also be discovered at autopsy on victims of severe burns and barotrauma and a number of other conditions ranging from diabetes to pancreatitis.

Air embolism

Air embolism is caused when a considerable volume of air gains access to the venous system and is carried to

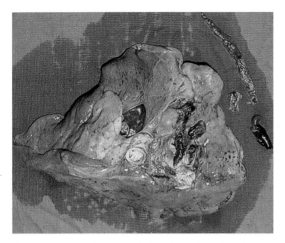

Figure 16.2 Fatal pulmonary emboli occluding the major pulmonary arteries 2 weeks after repair of a fractured femur.

the heart, where it fills the right atrium and ventricle with frothy bubbles. These bubbles are compressible and so cannot be pumped onward during systole and, as a result, they form an air lock, which causes circulatory failure. Air can gain access to the veins by a number of routes, including opening of the large veins in the neck following cutting of the throat or during operations such as thyroidectomy. The head must be above the level of the chest to cause a suction effect into the superior vena cava.

Another cause of air emboli is the use of a Higginson syringe to procure an abortion: air or frothy fluid is forced into the placental bed and enters the bloodstream. A different mechanism operates in decompression sickness in divers or high-altitude flyers, in which bubbles of nitrogen gas are formed in the blood. This may happen in any blood vessel in the body and clearly may result in direct effects on many organs, including the heart and brain.

The minimum volume of air needed to cause death from cardiac embolism is debatable, but is probably of the order of at least 100 mL in humans. Any gas that remains after absorption of oxygen by the erythrocytes (which will be mainly nitrogen) cannot penetrate the lung capillary bed to any extent, nor can it move upwards in the jugular veins against the blood flow. Therefore, 'cerebral air embolism' probably does not exist, and the descriptions and photographs of bubbles of gas in the cerebral veins are probably artefacts caused when the skull-cap is removed during autopsy.

Pulmonary thrombo-embolism

This is mentioned in Chapter 17 as a common cause of sudden death, but is also one of the most common consequences of injury of any type. After any significant tissue damage, there is an increase in the coagulability of the blood. If the injury results in immobility, this will have the effect of applying pressure on the calves of the legs, which in turn reduces the blood flow in the legs. These factors encourage thrombosis in the deep veins of the legs after any injury and many surgical operations. However, leg vein thrombosis may occur after any period of stagnation or pressure on the legs and it has been reported in long-distance air passengers (now called the Economy Class Syndrome) and even in those who sit in deck chairs for long periods.

Rarely, thromboses develop in other veins and form the source of pulmonary emboli, but the leg veins are overwhelmingly the most common focus. Pelvic vein thrombosis, even in association with pregnancy and childbirth, is less common than alleged.

Deep vein thromboses are extremely common, but most remain *in situ* and many patients are symptom free. The thromboses begin distally and spread proximally in the blood flow; they are most commonly found in the calves and may extend proximally as far as the saphenous, femoral or even iliac veins. Many thromboses spontaneously detach (in part or in whole) from the wall of the vein to form thrombo-emboli, which are swept off in the venous bloodstream to the right side of the heart. On leaving the heart, they encounter increasingly smaller vessels as the pulmonary arteries divide and, when the size of the embolus is equal to the size of the pulmonary artery, it can go no further and so it obstructs the vessel like a cork in a bottle. Pulmonary emboli may cause clinical symptoms of chest pain and haemoptysis or they may be silent. Larger emboli are commonly preceded by one or more smaller emboli. The large emboli may impact in the main trunk or in the large pulmonary arteries and cause rapid death.

The forensic significance of pulmonary emboli lies in their association with apparently non-fatal trauma. The victim, having survived the original injury, may even appear to be making an uncomplicated recovery, but suddenly collapses and dies some time later and pulmonary emboli are identified at the autopsy. About 80 per cent of fatal pulmonary emboli have a predisposing cause – trauma, surgical operation, immobility, childbirth etc. The remaining 20 per cent appear spontaneously with no previous warning, and unsuspected deep vein thrombosis in the legs is commonly found at autopsy.

Foreign-body embolism

Though rare, extrinsic foreign material sometimes gains entry to the veins and reaches the lungs. Most common these days is the contaminant material produced when tablets, intended for oral use and containing inert fillers (often starch), are crushed and injected and the particles of filler become impacted in the pulmonary capillaries. Other drugs used intravenously (heroin etc.) may be diluted or 'cut' with a variety of materials, including starch or talc, which are also insoluble and embolize in the lungs. Both starch and talc are doubly refractile materials under polarized light when viewed in histological sections and can be easily identified. This foreign material may, over time, provoke a response from the body and foreign-body granulomas may be seen.

Other, far more rare, foreign-body emboli include bullets and shotgun pellets, which may even be found in coronary or cerebral arteries and in other vital blood vessels. The use of cannulae and stents in modern medicine has resulted in rare cases of iatrogenic emboli. The clinical history is crucial to the understanding and interpretation of these cases.

Amniotic fluid embolism

This is a complication of labour in which there is escape of amniotic fluid into the maternal circulation, which can certainly provoke a fatal response by blocking the pulmonary capillaries in a similar fashion to fat emboli. Amniotic fluid is also known to be able to produce disseminated intravascular coagulation (DIC). Histological examination of multiple sections of lung using special staining methods for keratin squames is often needed to establish the diagnosis, which is usually suspected clinically. In addition to the amniotic fluid, fetal squames, lanugo, vernix lipoid and even meconium can be found in the maternal lungs in extreme cases.

DISSEMINATED INTRAVASCULAR COAGULATION

This condition results from a widespread activation of the clotting mechanisms, whether by exposure to tissue factors or phospholipids via activation of factor X (extrinsic pathway) or by activation of the factor XII cascade (intrinsic pathway). Many diverse things can initiate this abnormal coagulation reaction, but whatever the trigger, the result of this widespread activation of the clotting mechanism is that fibrin clots form throughout the vascular system. These clots obstruct the blood vessels and lead to ischaemia or infarction in skin and internal organs. When the clotting factors are consumed, bleeding may become widespread and there is an associated depletion of platelets as they attach to the fibrin clots. The fibrinolytic system is also activated so that, until the clotting factors and the fibrinolytic enzymes are consumed, there is a very real contest between the two sides of the haemostatic system.

DIC is usually diagnosed in life and can be confirmed at autopsy by the unusual amount and distribution of bleeding in the body and by the finding of fibrin clots and the signs of ischaemia or infarction of many organs on microscopy.

ADULT RESPIRATORY DISTRESS SYNDROME

This lung condition is a complication of a whole range of traumatic or stressful incidents, including aspiration of gastric contents, heavy impacts on the thorax, inhalation of irritant gases, pulmonary infections and systemic shock.

Clinically, the lungs become increasingly stiff and hard to ventilate and respiratory failure develops due to poor gas exchange. At autopsy, the stiff, oedematous lungs retain their shape even when removed from the chest cavity. Histologically, the intra-alveolar exudates, hyaline membranes and intrapulmonary haemorrhages of the acute phase later give way to cellular proliferation, which can become fibrotic if there is survival for long enough.

SUPRARENAL HAEMORRHAGE

A not uncommon, but rarely diagnosed, complication of injury is haemorrhage into the adrenal glands, which can sometimes be bilateral. It tends to occur a few days after severe trauma or infection. The bleeding, which is sometimes massive enough to expand the glands to several times their normal size, occurs in the medulla, with the cortex being stretched into a thin

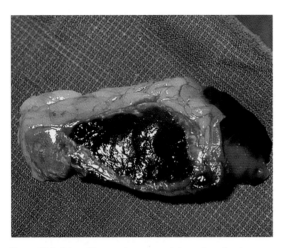

Figure 16.3 Adrenal haemorrhage several days after a head injury. The haemorrhage was bilateral and not related to abdominal trauma.

line around the haematoma. The bleeding is not due to direct mechanical damage, but appears to be neurologically mediated via the sympathetic nervous system, in much the same way as acute gastric erosions and subendocardial haemorrhage are related to parasympathetic over-activity. When associated with meningococcal infection, these bilateral adrenal haemorrhages form the typical Waterhouse–Friederichsen syndrome.

SUBENDOCARDIAL HAEMORRHAGES

Subendocardial haemorrhages are a non-specific finding in many cases of death following general trauma, particularly when it was associated with hypotension and following fatal head injuries. It is important that subendocardial haemorrhages are not confused with direct cardiac trauma in these cases.

LIVERPOOL
JOHN MOORES UNIVERSITY
AVRIL ROBARTS LRC
TITHEBARN STREET
LIVERPOOL L2 2ER
TEL. 0151 231 4022

Chapter seventeen

Unexpected and Sudden Death from Natural Causes

In countries where deaths have to be officially certified, the responsibility for certification falls either to the doctor who attended the patient during life or one who can reasonably be assumed to know sufficient of the clinical history to give a reasonable assessment of the cause of death. This is an 'honest opinion, fairly given', but many studies have shown that there is a large error rate in death certificates and that in 25–60 per cent of deaths there are significant differences between the clinician's presumption of the cause of death and the lesions or diseases actually displayed at the autopsy.

Unfortunately, it seems that there has been little or no improvement in the problems of certification of death over the years and as a result the raw epidemiological data gathered by national statistical bureaux must be treated with some caution. All doctors should take the task of certifying the cause of death very seriously but, regrettably, it is a job usually delegated to the most junior, and least experienced, member of the team. A review of death certification is currently being performed in the UK in the wake of the serial murders of Harold Shipman, a general practitioner in Manchester.

There is a different approach to sudden and unexpected deaths, as these deaths are usually reportable to the authorities for medico-legal investigation. In England and Wales, doctors should only issue a death certificate if they are satisfied that they know the cause of death and that it is definitely due to natural causes; additionally, they must have either examined the patient (alive) within the previous 14 days or they must have examined the body after death.

The World Health Organization (WHO) definition of a sudden death is within 24 hours of the onset of symptoms, but in forensic practice most sudden deaths occur within minutes or even seconds of the onset of symptoms. Indeed, it is very likely that a death that is delayed by hours will not be referred to the coroner or other medico-legal authority, as a diagnosis may well have been made, and a death certificate can be completed by the attending doctors.

It is crucial to remember that a sudden death is not necessarily unexpected and an unexpected death is not necessarily sudden, but these two facets are often combined.

CAUSES OF SUDDEN AND UNEXPECTED DEATH

When a natural death is very rapid, the cause is almost inevitably cardiovascular. Indeed, if a person collapses and is clinically dead before bystanders can assist, this can only be due to a cardiac event resulting in a cardiac arrest. Virtually no other mode of death operates so quickly. Extra-cardiac causes, even those elsewhere in the cardiovascular system, are rarely so rapidly fatal. Of course, in all such discussions of this nature, 'death' must be defined and, for our present purposes, irreversible cardiac arrest is taken as the criterion of death.

CARDIOVASCULAR SYSTEM

Disease of the heart

Most sudden unexpected deaths (SUDs) are caused by disease of the cardiovascular system. Although there is a huge geographical variation, due to the remarkable differences in the recorded incidence of atherosclerosis, the prime causes of SUD usually lies in the heart itself. The following lesions are the most obvious.

CORONARY ARTERY DISEASE

- Coronary stenosis from narrowing of the lumen by atheroma may lead to chronic ischaemia of the muscle supplied by that coronary vessel. If the myocardium becomes ischaemic, it may also become electrically unstable and liable to develop arrhythmias. The oxygen requirement of the myocardium is dependent upon the heart rate and so anything that increases the heart rate (exercise, a large meal or a sudden adrenaline response to stress or to anger, fear or other emotion) will lead to an increase in the oxygen requirements. If these cannot be met due to the restriction of the blood flow through the stenotic vessel, the myocardium distal to the stenosis will become ischaemic. There is no need for this ischaemia to produce a myocardial infarct; it just has to be sufficiently severe to initiate fatal arrhythmias and, if the region rendered ischaemic includes one of the pace-making nodes or a major branch of the conducting system, the risk that rhythm abnormalities will develop is greatly increased.
- Complications of atheromatous plaques may worsen the coronary stenosis and subsequent myocardial ischaemia. Bleeding may occur into a plaque and this can be seen as subintimal haemorrhage at autopsy. Sudden expansion of the plaque may lead to rupture, which may also occur if the plaque ulcerates. When a

plaque ruptures, the extruded cholesterol, fat and fibrous debris will be washed downstream in the coronary artery and impact distally, often causing multiple mini-infarcts. The endothelial cap of a ruptured plaque may act as a flap valve within the vessel and cause a complete obstruction.

An atheromatous plaque is a site for the development of mural thrombus, which will further reduce the vessel lumen without necessarily fully blocking the vessel.

- Coronary thrombosis is commonly over-diagnosed by clinicians as a cause of sudden death, and less than one-third of sudden cardiac deaths reveal macroscopic or microscopic evidence of coronary thrombus at autopsy. The simple stenosis and the complications of atheroma are both sufficient to cause death and much more common. However, coronary thrombosis is still a frequent finding at autopsy and it will be associated with an area of myocardial infarct, providing there has been a sufficiently long period of survival for the macroscopic changes of infarction to develop.
- Myocardial infarction occurs when there is severe stenosis or complete occlusion of a coronary artery so that the blood supply is insufficient to maintain the oxygenation of the myocardium. However, if there is adequate collateral circulation, blood can still reach the myocardium by other routes. The fatal effects of an infarct may appear at any time after the muscle has become ischaemic.
- The area of muscle damaged by a myocardial infarction is further weakened by the process of cellular death and the inflammatory response to these necrotic cells. The area of the myocardial infarct is weakest between 3 days and 1 week after the clinical onset of the infarct and it is at this time that the weakened area of myocardium may rupture and cause sudden death from a haemopericardium and cardiac tamponade. The rupture occasionally occurs through the interventricular septum, resulting in a left–right shunt. If a papillary muscle is infarcted, it may rupture, which will allow part of the mitral valve to prolapse, which may be associated with sudden death or may present as a sudden onset of valve insufficiency.
- An infarct heals by fibrosis, and fibrotic plaques in the wall of the ventricle or septum may interfere with physical or electrical cardiac function. Cardiac aneurysms may form at sites of infarction; they may calcify and they may rupture.

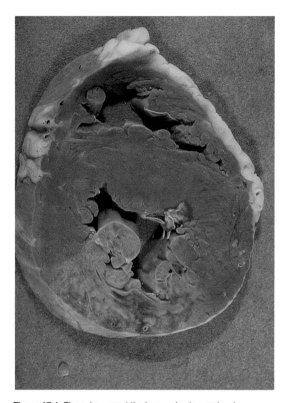

Figure 17.1 The paler area at the lower edge is a regional myocardial infarction of several days' duration.

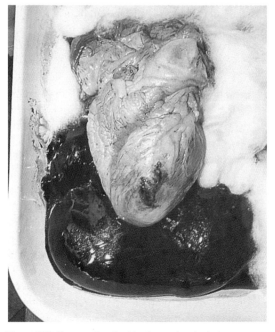

Figure 17.2 Haemopericardium due to a ruptured anterior myocardial infarct. Death was due to cardiac tamponade.

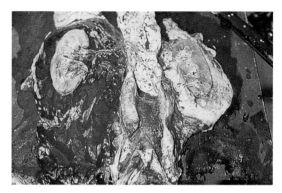

Figure 17.3 Ruptured atheromatous aortic aneurysm of the abdominal aorta causing massive retroperitoneal haemorrhage.

• Physical lesions in the cardiac conducting system have been studied intensively in recent years, especially in relation to sudden death. Many different abnormalities have been found, varying from extensive fibrosis to haemorrhage, tumours and infective lesions. It may be difficult to determine if such lesions are the cause of the fatal arrhythmia or merely an incidental finding, but in the absence of any other abnormality, it is reasonable to conclude that they were a significant factor in causing the death.

HYPERTENSIVE HEART DISEASE

This condition may lead to sudden cardiac death from left ventricular hypertrophy. The upper limit of normal heart weight is about 400 g (although this depends greatly on the body size and weight) and this may increase to 600 g or more, reflecting the increased thickness of the left ventricle. However, blood can only flow through the coronary arterioles during diastole because they are compressed during systole. At rest, when diastole is relatively long, the whole of the myocardium can be adequately perfused, but if the heart rate increases, diastolic time is reduced and the perfusion of the subendocardial cells is reduced. These cells become unstable and irritable and may produce arrhythmias and fibrillation. Atheroma is often associated with hypertension so that the enlarged heart may also be deprived of a normal blood flow in the major coronary vessels by the presence of atheromatous plaques and their complications.

AORTIC STENOSIS

Aortic stenosis is a disease that classically affects males over the age of 60 years with tricuspid aortic valves, but which may also be seen in younger people who have a congenital bicuspid aortic valve. The myocardial hypertrophy is similar to hypertension and it leads to left ventricular hypertrophy, which may, in some cases, produce heart weights of over 700 g.

In aortic stenosis, the perfusion problem is worsened by the narrow valve, which results in a lower pressure at the coronary ostia and hence in the coronary arteries. Sudden death is common in these patients.

SENILE MYOCARDIAL DEGENERATION

Senescence is a well-accepted concept in all animals, and few humans survive beyond 90–100 years. The cause of a sudden death in these elderly individuals can be very difficult to determine. The senile heart is small, the surface vessels are tortuous and the myocardium is soft and brown due to accumulated lipofuscins in the cells.

PRIMARY MYOCARDIAL DISEASE

These are much less common than the degenerative conditions described above and they commonly affect a significantly younger age group. Myocarditis occurs in many infective diseases, such as diphtheria and virus infections, including influenza, but the clinical complications and sudden death associated with the infection may occur some days or even weeks after the main clinical symptoms. Care must be taken in interpreting the histological appearances of small foci of myocarditis because isolated collections of lymphocytes may be identified in the myocardium of young adults who have died suddenly from trauma, suggesting that these foci are simply incidental findings. These foci used to be known as 'isolated Fiedler's myocarditis'. Other infective and inflammatory processes can also involve the myocardium, including disseminated sarcoidosis.

A more definite group of intrinsic cardiac diseases is the 'cardiomyopathies'. The initial descriptions referred to cardiomegaly with huge hearts of over 1000 g and asymmetric thickening of the ventricular walls in the hypertrophic, obstructive type of cardiomyopathy (HOCM) or dilatation of the chambers in congestive cardiomyopathy. Both types of the disease are usually associated with areas of disordered myocardial fibres. Extensive research has now shown that the cardiomyopathies are a much more complex group of primary myocardial diseases, commonly with a genetic background, which often do not show the typical macroscopic appearances described above. Right ventricular cardiomyopathy is now described and is associated with fatty infiltration of the wall of the right ventricle.

Other primary myocardial diseases or conduction defects, many of which are inheritable, are now described and include long QT syndrome, Brugada syndrome and catecholaminergic polymorphic ventricular tachycardia. The autopsy in these cases will be entirely negative but, as DNA techniques improve, diagnosis will be made in the laboratory rather than the mortuary.

Diseases of the arteries

The most common lesion of the arteries themselves that is associated with sudden death is the aneurysm. Several varieties must be considered as they are very commonly found in autopsies on SUDs.

ATHEROMATOUS ANEURYSM OF THE AORTA

These aneurysms are most commonly found in elderly males in the abdominal region of the aorta. They are formed when the elastic component of the aortic wall below an atheromatous plaque is damaged and the blood pressure is able to balloon the weakened wall. The aneurysms may be saccular (expanding to one side) or fusiform (cylindrical). The wall of the aneurysm is commonly calcified and the lumen is commonly lined by old laminated thrombus.

Many aneurysms remain intact and are found as an incidental finding at autopsy, but others eventually rupture. The rupture may be repaired surgically if diagnosed in time, but many individuals die too quickly for any help to be given. Because the aorta lies in the retroperitoneal space, that is where the bleeding is found; it usually lies to one side and may envelope the kidney. Rarely, the aneurysm itself, or the retroperitoneal haematoma, ruptures through the retroperitoneal tissues to cause a haemoperitoneum.

DISSECTING ANEURYSM OF THE AORTA

The damage caused by an atheromatous plaque can also result in the weakening of the aortic media, and a defect in the intima, usually also associated with the plaque, allows blood from the lumen to dissect into this weakened area of media. Once the dissection has started, the pressure of the influx of blood extends the dissection along the aortic wall. The commonest site

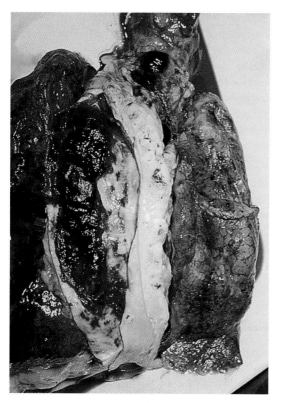

Figure 17.4 Dissecting thoracic aortic aneurysm. The true aortic lumen is to the right of the midline and the dissection lies to the left and is partly filled with adherent blood clot.

of origin of a dissecting aneurysm is in the thoracic aorta and the dissection usually tracks distally towards the abdominal region, sometimes reaching the iliac and even the femoral arteries. In fatal cases, the track may rupture at any point, resulting in haemorrhage into the thorax or abdomen. Alternatively, it can dissect proximally around the arch and into the pericardial sac, where it can produce a haemopericardium, cardiac tamponade and sudden death.

Dissecting aneurysms are also seen in association with diseases of the aortic media such as cystic medial degeneration.

SYPHILITIC ANEURYSMS

These are now relatively rare in Western countries due to the effective treatment of primary and secondary syphilis, but they are still encountered in routine autopsies on old people and in individuals from areas without an established health care system. The aneurysms are thin walled; they are most common in the thoracic

aorta and especially in the arch. They may rupture, causing torrential haemorrhage.

Intracranial vascular lesions

Several types of intracranial vascular lesions are important in sudden or unexpected death.

RUPTURED BERRY ANEURYSM

A relatively common cause of sudden collapse and often rapid death of young to middle-aged men and women is a subarachnoid haemorrhage resulting from rupture of a 'congenital' (berry) aneurysm of the basal cerebral arteries either in the circle of Willis itself or in the arteries which supply it. Whether berry aneurysms can be described as 'congenital' depends on the interpretation of the word: strictly speaking, they are not present at birth, but the weakness in the media of the vessel wall (usually at a bifurcation) from which they develop is present at birth. The aneurysms may be a few millimetres in diameter or they may extend to several centimetres; they may be single or multiple and they may be found on one or more arteries.

The aneurysms may be clinically silent or they may leak, producing a severe headache, neck stiffness, unconsciousness and sometimes paralysis or other neurological symptoms. The rupture of a berry aneurysm on the arterial circle of Willis allows blood to flood over the base of the brain or, if the aneurysm is embedded in the brain, into the brain tissue itself. The speed of death can be such that the initial impression is of a cardiac event. It is thought that sudden exposure of the brainstem to blood under arterial pressure depresses the cardiorespiratory centres in the brainstem.

The role of direct trauma in the rupture of an aneurysm is in dispute. It seems reasonable to suspect that a large, fragile aneurysm on the circle of Willis might be damaged by a substantial head injury; such an aneurysm should be easy to identify at autopsy and so this should not present a diagnostic problem. However, for the more common, small aneurysms situated deeply inside the skull, it seems unlikely that a blow that causes no other cranial or intracranial injury would cause the aneurysm to be selectively ruptured.

There is another cause for subarachnoid haemorrhage that is well known to be associated with trauma to the head and neck following violence or an assault when there is forceful lateral flexion of the neck or rotation of the head. The anatomical course of the vertebral arteries is convoluted and, for much of their course in the neck, they are protected within the lateral foramina of the cervical vertebrae. However, they are more exposed to trauma above the first cervical vertebra, and it has been claimed that most traumatic subarachnoid haemorrhages are due to tearing of this extra-cranial region of a vertebral artery within or adjacent to the first cervical vertebra or between it and the base of the skull. Damage to the vertebral arteries at these sites requires the bleeding to dissect in the wall of the artery as far as the base of the skull and then rupture to cause the subarachnoid haemorrhage. This dissection in the arterial wall can often be identified more easily than the intimal damage that marks the origin of the haemorrhage. There may be bruising on the skin surface of the neck to indicate direct trauma or the bruising may be confined to the deep muscles of the neck, indicating indirect trauma to the neck.

Cerebral haemorrhage

Sudden bleeding into the brain substance is common, usually in old age and in those with significant

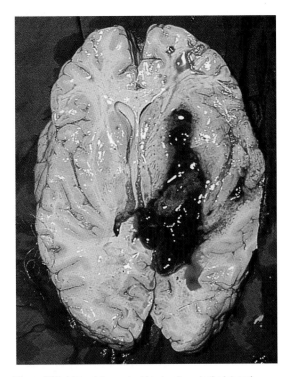

Figure 17.5 A large intracerebral haemorrhage in the internal capsule, with extension into the ventricle.

hypertension, and together with cerebral thrombosis and the resulting infarction, this is the commonest cause of the well-recognized cluster of neurological signs colloquially termed a 'stroke'.

Spontaneous intracerebral haemorrhage is most often found in the external capsule of one hemisphere and arises from rupture of a micro-aneurysm of the lenticulo-striate artery, sometimes called a Charcot–Bouchard aneurysm. The sudden expansion of a haematoma compresses the internal capsule and may destroy some of it, leading to a hemiplegia.

Haemorrhage can also occur in the cerebellum and the mid-brain, possibly as a result of a ruptured aneurysm or other vascular abnormality, although the abnormality may be extremely difficult to identify at autopsy. Death is seldom instantaneous, although it can be extremely rapid following a haemorrhage in the brainstem.

CEREBRAL THROMBOSIS AND INFARCTION

Cerebral thrombosis rarely causes sudden death, as the process of infarction is relatively slow, although the neurological symptoms and signs may have a very rapid onset and be severe.

The term 'cerebrovascular accident' (CVA) is in common usage, both as a clinical diagnosis and as a cause of death. Occasionally, it is misinterpreted by the public, and sometimes also by legal officials, as indicating an unnatural cause of death because of the use of the word 'accident'. To avoid this small risk, it is much more satisfactory, if the exact cause is known, to use the specific term that describes the aetiology – 'cerebral haemorrhage' or 'cerebral infarction' – or, if the aetiology is not known, to use the generic term 'cerebrovascular lesion'.

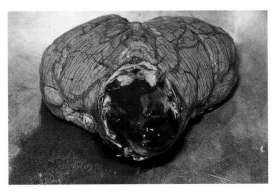

Figure 17.6 Pontine haemorrhage in a hypertensive individual.

RESPIRATORY SYSTEM

The major cause of sudden death within the respiratory organs is again vascular. Pulmonary embolism is very common and, in fact, is the most clinically under-diagnosed cause of death. In almost every case, the source of the emboli is in the leg veins. Tissue trauma, especially where it is associated with immobility or bed rest, is a very common predisposing factor in the development of deep vein thrombosis. Most thromboses remain silent and cause no problems, but a proportion embolize and block pulmonary arteries of varying size. Some produce no lung lesions at all, whereas others produce infarcts that may or may not lead to clinical signs, and a minority (though an appreciable number) block a major vessel and cause death.

About 80 per cent of pulmonary embolism deaths have a predisposing cause such as fractures, tissue trauma, surgical operation, bed rest, forced immobility etc., but the remainder occur unexpectedly in normal, ambulant people who have reported no clinical symptoms. This makes establishing the relationship of death to an injurious event difficult. For the purposes of civil law (where 'the balance of probabilities' is enough), the embolism can often be linked to the trauma, but in a criminal trial in which the higher standard of proof – 'beyond reasonable doubt' – is required, it is much harder to relate fatal pulmonary emboli to the trauma.

Other rare causes of sudden death in the respiratory system include a massive haemoptysis from cavitating pulmonary tuberculosis or from a malignant tumour. Rapid (but not sudden) deaths can also occur from fulminating chest infections, especially virulent forms of influenza.

GASTROINTESTINAL SYSTEM

Once again, the causes of sudden death have a vascular component in that very severe bleeding from a gastric or duodenal peptic ulcer can be fatal in a short time, but, more commonly, the bleeding is less torrential and is therefore amenable to medical or surgical treatment. Mesenteric thrombosis and embolism, usually related to aortic or more generalized atheroma, may result in infarction of the gut, but, once again, a rapid but not sudden death is expected if the infarction remains undiagnosed.

Perforation of a peptic ulcer can be fatal in hours if not treated and intestinal infarction due to a strangulated hernia or obstruction due to torsion of the bowel around an area of peritoneal adhesions can also be fulminating and fatal conditions, as can peritonitis arising from diverticular disease or a perforated carcinoma. Many of these conditions present as sudden death in elderly people because they cannot or will not seek assistance at the onset of the symptoms and are then unable to do so as their condition worsens.

GYNAECOLOGICAL CONDITIONS

When a woman of childbearing age is found unexpectedly dead, a complication of pregnancy must be considered to be the most likely cause of her death until all such causes are excluded. Abortion remains one possibility anywhere in the world, but especially in countries where illegal abortion is still very common (see Chapter 19).

A ruptured ectopic pregnancy, which is usually tubal in position, is another grave obstetric emergency that can end in death from intraperitoneal bleeding unless rapidly treated by surgical intervention.

As a 'rule of thumb', the three commonest causes of death in a woman of reproductive age are:

1 a natural complication of pregnancy such as ruptured ectopic gestation or an induced complication such as an abortion;
2 pulmonary embolism from leg vein thrombosis;
3 ruptured cerebral aneurysm.

DEATHS FROM ASTHMA AND EPILEPSY

In both conditions, death may occur during an attack and the autopsy will reveal specific features to enable a positive diagnosis to be made. However, both of these conditions are also associated with a few sudden and unexpected deaths each year where the specific features of an attack are absent and for which no obvious cause of death can be identified at autopsy.

Even well-controlled epileptic patients may die rapidly and inexplicably; it was once thought that they must have been exhausted from status epilepticus, but this is now not thought to be so. There are some who doubt that these patients are even having a fit when they die because of the lack of pathological features, but many epileptics have fits that leave no pathological signs, rendering this theory unlikely. Epileptics are also at risk from the hazards of all types of accidents during a pre-fit aura (if they have one), while having a fit or immediately afterwards; these hazards include falls, drowning, suffocation and postural asphyxia.

Bronchial asthma is also associated with rare unexplained sudden and unexpected deaths, even where there is no evidence of status asthmaticus or even of an unusually severe or prolonged asthmatic episode. Several decades ago, an increase in sudden deaths in asthmatics was traced to the over-use of adrenergic drugs – especially the self-administered dose given by inhaler – but awareness amongst doctors soon reduced this hazard.

Chapter eighteen

Sexual Offences

TYPES OF SEXUAL OFFENCE

Though the legal definitions of particular sexual offences will vary from country to country, the classification of illegal sexual acts or actions is relatively standard, even though the names of the various offences may differ. The following list is from English law but can be modified for other jurisdictions.

Rape

Rape is the most serious sexual offence. It can only be committed by a biological male, but the victim can be of either sex. Rape was re-defined in the Criminal Justice and Public Order Act (1994) as 'non-consensual penetration of the vagina or the anus by a penis'. Consent is crucial and the act is rape if the man either knows that the victim does not consent to the act of intercourse or is reckless (unconcerned) as to whether they consent or not. This provision replaces the old terminology of 'fear, force or fraud' because any consent given under any of those circumstances would not be valid. The same will apply if alcohol or drugs are used to render the individual unconscious and also to intercourse with a sleeping individual.

The law in England and Wales does not distinguish between an act between strangers and one between those with a relationship, legal or otherwise, and it is now possible for a man to be convicted of raping his wife. The law only applies to boys over the age of 14 years, because English law presumes that a boy under that age is incapable of rape. This is medically untrue but cannot be challenged in England, although it may in Scotland.

Sexual intercourse is no longer part of the definition of rape, having been replaced by the term 'penetration'. The use of this term reflects the legal

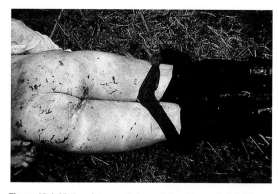

Figure 18.1 Victim of rape and strangulation. Removal of clothing, bleeding from the perineum and soiling of the skin can be seen.

definition of sexual intercourse previously applied, which was any degree of penile insertion, even if this is only just between the labia or just into the anal margin. Neither full penetration nor ejaculation is necessary and, in terms of vaginal rape, the rupture of the hymen is irrelevant.

Individuals with substantial mental disease or deficiency that could be defined as 'severe mental impairment' under the Mental Health Act of 1983 cannot give valid consent to sexual intercourse, whatever their age.

Unlawful sexual intercourse

In Britain, the age of consent to heterosexual intercourse is 16 years, but it is different in other countries, for instance in some states of the USA it is 18 years. Below that age a girl cannot give legal consent for sexual intercourse and hence any act of intercourse is always 'unlawful'. Sexual intercourse in these circumstances is termed 'unlawful sexual intercourse' and it is a charge that is, in essence, divided into separate offences depending on the age of the girl and the man.

If the girl is under 13 years of age, this offence is the same as rape and it is immaterial if consent was given or not. The maximum penalty for this offence is life imprisonment.

If the girl is over 13 but under 16 years of age, a man can avoid conviction in England and Wales if:

a. (i) he is under 24 years of age **and**
   (ii) he has never have been charged with a similar offence previously **and**
   (iii) he believed that the girl was over 16 **and**

(iv) he had reasonable cause for that belief due to her appearance, dress, make-up and behaviour etc.

or

b. he believed her to be his lawful wife.

Indecent assault

Indecent assault covers a very wide spectrum of acts or actions performed by members of either sex on victims of either sex. These acts may range from a failed attempt at penile penetration of the vagina or anus, to the actual penetration of the vagina or anus with a finger or an object, to penetration of the mouth by the penis (forced fellatio), to touching or fondling of the buttocks, breasts, thighs, perineum, penis or putting a hand up a woman's skirt or inside a man's trousers. Only the more serious, penetrative forms of indecent assault are likely to have physical medical aspects unless other injuries are caused during the incident such as bruises, bite marks and abrasions. All the acts are very likely to leave the victims psychologically traumatized.

Indecent exposure

Indecent exposure, often known colloquially as 'flashing', occurs when a person, usually a man, displays his genitals in public to the annoyance and embarrassment of members of the public. This is physically harmless to victims but may cause them psychological distress. Restraint and psychiatric treatment of the offender are probably more important than a custodial sentence.

Indecency with children

More serious are the men and women who prey on small children, not to assault or touch them or their genitalia, but to encourage the child to handle or masturbate the offender's sexual organs. In England and Wales, a special law was passed in 1960 (Indecency with Children Act) to make this behaviour illegal with a child below 14 years of age; this closed a loop-hole in the Sexual Offences Act of 1956.

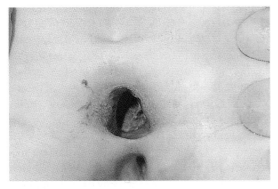

Figure 18.2 Anal penetration of a young child with dilatation, abrasion, marginal tearing and skin tags. Dilatation alone is insufficient for a firm diagnosis of buggery.

Incest

Incest is not universally considered to be a criminal offence; indeed, it was (and is) a socially acceptable part of normal behaviour in some cultures. The most common situation occurs when a father has sexual intercourse with his own teenage daughter when his wife was in the later stages of pregnancy or in the puerperium. In some countries and religions, even from ancient times, it was recognized that there were genetic risks attached to births arising from the mating of close relations, and from the Biblical period onward lists of 'prohibited degrees' of relationships were declared.

The extent of these lists varies from country to country and even between religious and secular codes in the same country. In Britain the law forbids marriage or penile/vaginal sexual intercourse between a man and a woman he knows to be his mother, daughter, grand-daughter, sister or half-sister; a similar list of exclusions exists for the female side. Both the man and the woman are liable to prosecution for such an act. Other sexual acts between relations are covered by other laws and, if truly consensual, they do not constitute an offence.

Doctors, especially family practitioners, may be the first to learn of incest in a family and if one participant is a child, they must act immediately to prevent any further acts of incest and to treat the child physically and psychologically. If pregnancy or sexually transmitted diseases are diagnosed, the child must be referred to specialists for treatment.

There is a range of further options open to doctors in socially advanced countries and they must decide how best to respond, but there is no doubt that the doctor's over-riding duty is to the welfare of the child. The doctor may decide to involve the police immediately or may decide to take professional advice from a counselling organization such as the National Society for the Prevention of Cruelty to Children (or the equivalent in other countries), the Social Services Department of the city or county authority or possibly from a senior paediatrician at a local hospital. Whatever the decision, the doctor should keep full notes of all telephone calls, conversations or other communications with professional organizations and the police as well as with the child and his or her parents.

When incest occurs between adult relatives, the situation is far more difficult, as legally the woman (or man) is a free agent and it might be thought that she could remove herself from the relationship. However, in practice, this is seldom an easy option for her and, in fact, the relationship is often more abusive than simply incestuous and requests for assistance must be treated very seriously, irrespective of the wishes of other members of the family.

Bestiality

Bestiality is sexual intercourse with animals, either vaginal or anal. This includes all animals, including birds, the usual victims being pets and farm animals, which are sometimes tortured and killed in the process. Though doctors are rarely involved in the investigation of this offence, they may sometimes be asked to examine genital injuries or infections in a man or woman that have been sustained in one of these acts. Veterinary surgeons and forensic scientists are more commonly involved in relation to injuries to animals and in the detection and identification of animal secretions and hairs found on a suspect and human semen in the animal. Though bestiality is more common than usually thought, especially in the countryside, few prosecutions are ever brought.

Homosexual offences

In many countries, all sexual acts between men are illegal and the penalties may be severe. In England and Wales, the Sexual Offences Act (1967) allowed for homosexual acts in private between consenting males over the age of 21 years, but with the specific exclusion of members of the armed forces or merchant seamen. The age of consent has now been reduced to 18 years and there is considerable pressure to reduce it further to 16 to match the heterosexual age of consent for females. In Scotland and Ireland, no such act was introduced, but prosecutions are now rarely if ever brought. Homosexual acts between females ('lesbianism') have never been a criminal offence unless they offend against public decency.

Under the terms of the 1967 act, anal intercourse between consenting males is not an offence, but anal intercourse with a woman or a boy over the age of 16 but below the minimum age stipulated in the act is always an offence whether they consent or not. Oral or manual stimulation has never been an offence under English law provided it is not performed in public. The redefinition of rape now allows for male rape and, like vaginal rape, proof of anal penetration by the penis has to be provided, though ejaculation of semen is not relevant to the offence.

THE GENUINENESS OF ALLEGATIONS OF SEXUAL ASSAULT

Doctors of either sex are at particular risk of the allegations of patients that they have been indecently assaulted during the course of a consultation, examination or treatment. The allegation may range from improper touching to kissing, fondling the breasts or genitalia and even actual intercourse. If substantiated, doctors are very likely to lose their medical registration after disciplinary proceedings and it is increasingly likely that they will also face a criminal prosecution.

However, some of the allegations made by patients are false – but this will not lessen the distress felt by doctors and their families while the allegations are investigated. All of which makes it imperative that, wherever possible, and certainly when performing intimate examinations or giving an anaesthetic in a doctor's or dentist's surgery (now not an approved process), the practitioner should have a chaperone (preferably of the same sex as the patient) in the same room. This may be extremely difficult in family practice, particularly when doctors have to carry out house calls on their own.

Though reliable statistics are very hard to obtain, the trend in the reporting of sexual crimes to the police suggests that less than one-fifth are reported to, and hence investigated by, the police. It is claimed that at least part of this under-reporting is because women know that they will have to undergo questioning by the police, an intimate medical examination and court appearances and they also fear a possible attack upon their character by defence lawyers. It is to be hoped that the changes in both the police and the medical investigations of rape and other sexual assaults, together with the changes in the processes and attitudes of the courts, will dispel some of these fears. Any victim of a sexual offence will have been violently traumatized and will need all of the support that can be provided to overcome their fears of the criminal justice system.

FORENSIC EXAMINATION OF VICTIMS OF SEXUAL OFFENCES

This is a highly specialized area of clinical forensic medicine and the following notes are intended as outline guidance only. A detailed text of clinical forensic medicine should be consulted for more detail if necessary. The examination of both the victim and perpetrator will be needed.

Ideally, the examination needs to be performed as soon as possible after the incident, but this is not always possible due to delayed reporting by the victim or simply because the victim does not feel able to be examined; the victim's need are obviously paramount. Examination of the victim (or the accused) must be performed in a suitable and well-equipped room, which may now be a specially constructed suite at a police station or hospital or in a medical room at the police station or possibly in a hospital casualty department. Wherever the examination is to be performed, there must be a guarantee of privacy for the individual who is to be examined, and adequate lighting and other facilities for the doctor performing the examination. The victim may wish to have a friend or relative present during the examination and the carer of a child will almost certainly need to be present.

It is imperative that informed consent is obtained and that the doctor explains the limits of confidentiality of this examination. In particular, the doctor must explain that no absolute guarantee of confidentiality can be given because he may be ordered by a court to disclose anything that is said or seen during the course of the examination; this applies equally to the victim and the accused. The individual must be aware that he or she can stop the examination at any time.

The victim will normally have been interviewed by the police or other legal officer to ascertain the sequence of events and the acts that were committed. In these circumstances it is seldom necessary for the examining doctor to obtain the detailed history of the events again, as the main facts can be provided by the interviewing officer. The doctor can, if necessary, ask the victim some additional questions in order to clarify particular aspects.

A relevant medical and sexual history will need to be taken, which should include details of any pre-existing conditions or behavioural pattern that may have an influence on any physical findings during the examination.

The physical examination will commence with a general examination concentrating on evidence of injury and disease, and all abnormalities should be noted and the injuries described and measured. Samples of head hair and fingernails, blood and urine should be obtained. The specific anogenital examination should be performed last and the extent of the examination will depend on each individual case; for instance if only fellatio is alleged, there is probably no need for a full anogenital examination.

The examination of the anogenital region of the victim will specifically include examination for congenital abnormalities and diseases as well as for evidence of injury. In all cases, combings of the pubic hair and retrieval of any foreign objects from the region are essential.

Unless some sharp object is used during a sexual assault, the injuries that will be found, if any, are those of blunt trauma caused by digital or penile trauma. Occasionally, injuries associated with 'fisting' or the use of an object may be seen.

Examination of the female anogenital region should commence with examination of the labia for injuries; two dry swabs are taken at this time. The vagina is then examined using a clean speculum and any foreign material such as lubricant, condoms or other objects are recovered and retained for forensic scientific examination. The walls of the vagina are carefully examined for injury, which may, rarely, include penetration by either blunt or sharp force. The hymen is examined and the general appearance and any evidence of recent injury including tears are recorded. The relevance of hymenal injuries is greatest in the young and the sexually inexperienced, but any injuries must be interpreted with great care. High vaginal and endocervical swabs are taken and low vaginal swabs are taken when the speculum is removed. Colposcopic examination of the female genital tract is advocated by many, but not all, forensic practitioners. However, this specialist equipment is expensive and may only be available in specialist rape examination suites or in hospital gynaecology departments.

Examination of the penis includes documentation of any congenital or acquired abnormalities and evidence of infection or foreign bodies in, on or around the genital area. A thorough search for injuries should be performed, including retraction of the foreskin to examine the glans in the uncircumcized male. Swabs of the shaft and of the glans may be taken and, in the dead victim, urethral swabs may also be obtained.

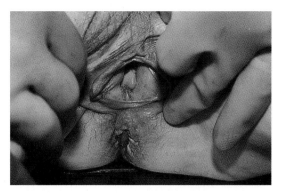

Figure 18.3 Suspected vaginal intercourse with an older woman. There is reddening and abrasion of the lower vagina but, in the absence of semen, manual penetration may be the cause. Infection must be excluded.

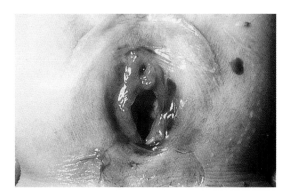

Figure 18.4 Vaginal rape of a small child with swelling, reddening and a posterior tear of the vulva.

The examination of the anus is the same for both sexes. After examination for congenital and acquired abnormalities and diseases, swabs should be taken from the perianal region, the anal canal and the lower rectum, and foreign material, including lubricant, condoms or other objects, should be swabbed or recovered. The anus, anal canal and rectum should then be inspected for injury, using a proctoscope if this will be tolerated by the individual. Damage to the anal mucosa may be referred to by a number of different names, including fissures, tears or lacerations. It is important to remember that damage to the anus may be the result of factors other than direct trauma.

EXAMINATION OF AN ALLEGED ASSAILANT

If someone is arrested for a sexual offence, a medical examination is essential. However, the informed consent of the individual is still needed in most countries. The accused may wish to have a legal representative present and these wishes should be accommodated. The doctor will need to take, and to make a note of, a general history of the events as given by the perpetrator and also their general medical and social history, and the limitations of confidentiality must be explained clearly, as with the victims of a sexual assault.

A general examination of the body for signs of any injuries is essential. If there has been a struggle, the perpetrator may have received injuries, and groups of linear parallel scratches on the face, neck and chest from the victim's fingernails are not uncommon. Examination of the anogenital region rarely reveals any significant signs, although there may be some non-specific tenderness and reddening. Exceptionally, the glans or prepuce may be bruised and the frenum of the penis damaged, and faecal material may be recovered if anal penetration has been achieved. The use of Lugol's iodine test is now redundant: the idea was that iodine solution painted on to the glans would reveal the presence of vaginal squames by turning them brown due to the glycogen contained in the vaginal cells.

The recovery of trace evidence is often more important than the genital inspection. Samples of pubic hair should be taken, along with head and even moustache or beard hair if appropriate. The pubic hair should be combed out to recover foreign hairs or fibres. Blood samples for grouping, alcohol and DNA are taken and any evidence of venereal infection noted.

In small boys and children, damage to the anal ring is more likely than in older victims, though caution is needed in assessing anal size, especially in the dead, in whom post-mortem dilatation can be marked. In extreme cases, tearing of the mucosa may be seen. In older habitual homosexuals, the anus may be permanently dilated, with loss of sphincter tone and exposure of the anal mucosa. The older description of a 'funnel-shaped anus' with keratinization and thickening of the external skin is a rare phenomenon, but some silvery scaliness of the skin can occur adjacent to the anus from repeated penetration.

Chapter nineteen

Pregnancy and Abortion

There are a large number of medico-legal aspects of the reproductive years in the life of a female. In many countries, there are laws governing some aspects of virginity, conception, contraception, the pregnancy itself and the legal and illegal means of ending a pregnancy. There are considerable geographical and geopolitical variations in both the ethical and the legal attitudes of different countries and religions to each of these aspects.

CONCEPTION: ARTIFICIAL INSEMINATION, *IN-VITRO* FERTILIZATION AND EMBRYO RESEARCH

In recent years considerable ethical and legal problems have arisen because of the development of medical techniques of initiating pregnancy other than by sexual intercourse. There is great legal, moral and religious controversy over these matters and opinions vary widely from country to country and from religion to religion. Some countries have introduced legislation to ban or to control these practices, while others have not. In the UK, the Human Fertilization and Embryology Act (1990) sought to place all of these techniques, but particularly *in-vitro* fertilization and research on embryos, into a legal framework.

The techniques of assisted conception are now so extensive and in many cases so complex that they lie outside the scope of this textbook. In short, the techniques range from relatively simple techniques of artificial insemination using the sperm of either the partner or an anonymous donor through to the *in-vitro* fertilization of eggs that have been harvested from the mother or an egg donor with sperm donated by the father or a donor. The resulting fetus is then re-implanted at a very early stage of development into the uterus, which has been artificially prepared by exogenous hormones.

The ethical and religious conflicts that are generated by these new techniques are immense and, while some of the legal implications have been resolved in the UK, there is no doubt that as the research pushes at the boundaries of science and societies around the world re-evaluate their positions, there will be many other dilemmas that will need to be resolved.

PREGNANCY

It may be important, legally, to prove or disprove a current or a recent pregnancy for a number of reasons, which may include the following.

- Where a criminal abortion has been alleged, it may be necessary to prove that the woman had recently been pregnant.

- In some civil disputes about the estate of a dead husband, the pregnancy of the wife may affect the disposition of property.
- Women in advanced pregnancy may be excused attendance as a witness in a court: in those countries that still have capital punishment, the pregnancy of a convicted woman may postpone or cancel her execution.
- In charges of infanticide or concealment of birth, it may be relevant to show that the woman had recently been pregnant.
- For a variety of reasons, pregnancy may be a pretence and medical evidence may be required to disprove the condition.

Many of the reasons previously advanced for a clinical medical examination to determine the fact of, or the duration of, a pregnancy in an attempt to establish paternity have now been superseded by DNA analysis of the fetus or the baby and of the putative father(s). More recently, DNA has also been used to establish maternity and a woman has been charged with infanticide.

Evidence of pregnancy consists of both clinical signs and biochemical testing. Biochemical tests on urine for pregnancy-related hormones are now so sophisticated and accurate that they are sensitive enough to be reliably positive as early as a week or so after conception.

Clinical signs in the first trimester include breast swelling and tenderness, changes in the nipples, amenorrhoea, frequency of micturition, (inconstant) nausea, leucorrhoea, softening of the cervix and ballotment of the uterus on vaginal examination (Hegar's sign). Ultrasound scanning can identify pregnancy as early as 4 weeks.

Later in pregnancy, the uterine enlargement extends over the pelvic brim; palpation of the fetus is possible at about 16 weeks and palpation of fetal parts and the detection of fetal heart sounds are possible at about 24 weeks. Fetal movements may be detected and radiological and ultrasonic evidence of the fetus can be easily obtained.

Evidence of a recent or past pregnancy and of parturition may be needed for medico-legal purposes, in the living or the dead. No single feature is diagnostic, but the presence of groups of features may allow for an accurate assessment. Following a recent vaginal delivery there will be dilatation and laxity of the vaginal introitus, sometimes associated with perineal damage or evidence of an episiotomy. The uterus remains palpable above the symphysis pubis for up to 2 weeks.

A vaginal discharge (lochia) may be bloodstained for a few days and then brown for a week or more. The breast changes will depend on whether feeding is established, discontinued or suppressed by hormones. Whatever the ultimate appearance, immediately after delivery the breasts will be swollen and tense and will often have prominent surface veins. Milk will be expressible after the second or third day. The nipple and areolae will be darkened, a change that is nonspecific but that may persist in some degree almost permanently.

On the abdomen, the stretch marks (striae gravidarum), which are pink in late pregnancy and around the time of delivery, become paler with time and, after a year or so, eventually appear as white scars (lineae albicantes). The cervix remains dilated and soft for some time and may show a tear, which eventually forms a scar. The breast changes subside with the cessation of breast-feeding but the nipple darkening may persist, especially in dark-complexioned women. The remains of the hymen will either vanish completely or remain only as small remnants (carunculae mytriformes) and there is inconstant loss of the rugosity of the vaginal walls seen in virgins.

The normal duration of pregnancy is about 40 weeks or 280 days, though there is naturally no minimum period. The maximum duration of pregnancy is disputed, but medically it is unlikely to extend for more than 42–43 weeks. Legal decisions that pregnancy may extend to 350 days or more are medically untenable and were probably introduced to associate a pregnancy with the last known intercourse with the husband. In Nigeria, a claim that a pregnancy had 'lain dormant' for a number of years was accepted by a religious court; it is doubtful that such a claim would have been accepted elsewhere. The problems of paternity are now easily resolved by the use of DNA profiles, although these tests are expensive and may not be available throughout the world.

ABORTION

A considerable proportion of pregnancies fail to proceed to full term. About 20 per cent of known pregnancies fail and it is estimated that many others have failed so early that pregnancy is not even recognized. After a pregnancy is apparent, the loss of the fetus up to 24 weeks is usually called a 'spontaneous abortion' or 'miscarriage'; from 24 weeks to full term, it may be called a 'premature birth'. However, these temporal definitions are not universally accepted.

In addition to the spontaneous (natural) abortions, abortions may also be induced and these induced abortions may be therapeutic or criminal, depending on the circumstances and the prevailing law of the country in which the abortion occurs.

Criminal abortion

A criminal abortion is the deliberate ending of a pregnancy outside any legal provisions that have been made by the state for this act. In most countries, performing a criminal abortion is a serious criminal offence and, in addition to any criminal conviction, it would form grounds for the strict disciplining of any doctor who was shown to be involved.

Before the introduction of legal abortion in Britain in 1967, it was thought that between 40 and 80 per cent of all reported abortions were deliberately induced, either by the woman herself or by another person. The introduction of easily available and reliable contraception has reduced the number of unwanted pregnancies, and the introduction of legal abortion in many parts of the world has greatly reduced the morbidity and mortality from criminal abortion, as it has allowed for state control of the conditions under which abortions are performed and for control of the training and skills of the operators performing them.

There is continual pressure throughout the world for the repeal of liberal abortion laws, and counter-movements motivated by politics or religion may again restrict or even abolish legal termination of pregnancy. There is no doubt that the inevitable result of the abolition of legal abortion will be increased work for the gynaecologist and pathologist in dealing with a revival of criminal abortion and with the diseases, disability and deaths that will travel in its wake.

Where no provisions exist for legal abortions, women are still at the mercy of 'back-street abortionists', who are sometimes doctors, nurses or midwives but whose methods may be as unsatisfactory as their premises and instruments. Alternatively, an abortion may be induced by the woman herself – in some places this is said to be a common practice amounting almost to regular birth control.

Nearly all criminal abortions used to take place in the second or third month of pregnancy, when the woman could be certain that the missed periods and morning sickness had confirmed her pregnancy. The increasing use of sophisticated 'do-it-yourself' pregnancy tests in many countries will allow for earlier diagnosis of pregnancy and may result in earlier attendance for abortion.

THE DOCTOR'S ACTIONS IN RESPECT OF ILLEGAL ABORTIONS

Unless the law of the country allows termination of pregnancy, albeit sometimes only in specific and very limited circumstances, no doctor may abort a woman for any reason; as noted above, a criminal conviction and loss of medical registration may follow such an act. Where the law of a country does allow for therapeutic abortion, doctors with strong religious or moral objections to abortion cannot be forced by their terms of employment or contractual obligations to perform or assist in any termination of pregnancy. Even where abortion is permitted by law, doctors cannot be forced to take part in this act, but neither should they obstruct a patient wishing to obtain an abortion, but should instead refer her to a doctor who will be willing to assist her.

When a doctor learns that a criminal abortion has taken place, his obligations depend on the circumstances. If the act was performed by the woman herself, the doctor should confine himself to giving all necessary medical care, but it is not part of his duty to report the fact to the police or anyone else unless death occurs, in which case he is naturally obliged to notify the coroner or whatever other legal authority investigates unnatural deaths.

Unless doctors feel that their duty to the public over-rides their duty of confidentiality to their patient, they should not divulge the matter unless the woman gives her consent for them to do so. The law has sometimes thought otherwise, as in Britain in 1914, when a judge said that, 'The desire for a doctor to preserve confidentiality must be subordinated to the duty which is cast upon every good citizen to assist in the investigation of a serious crime'. The British Medical Association and the Royal College of Physicians took legal advice and resolved that, 'A medical practitioner should not under any circumstances disclose voluntarily, without the patient's consent, information obtained from that patient in the course of professional duties'. This is to be supported, but it must be remembered that the doctor has a duty of confidentiality to the patient and not to the abortionist, whose name, if known, could be disclosed to the police or other authority without any breach of confidentiality.

METHODS OF PERFORMING ILLEGAL ABORTION

The common methods of abortion vary greatly from country to country and range from semi-magical folk remedies to the sophisticated clinical methods identical to those used during a legal abortion. The following are the most common means of procuring abortion; however, few of them will be seen in countries with legal abortion laws.

Drugs and toxins have been used for millennia to try to remove unwanted pregnancies, but most of them are quite ineffective. In Western countries, the long list of substances formerly documented in forensic textbooks is of historical interest only. However, in developing countries, many folk medicines and more drastic poisons may be encountered, including a host of vegetable compounds such as juniper, pennyroyal, savin, rue, colocynth and aloes. In South-East Asia, unripe pineapple is alleged to produce miscarriage. However, none of these substances is known to have any predictable or significant effect on the uterus and they are often sold to exploit distressed women.

Other substances that have a contractile effect on smooth muscle have a better theoretical chance of success and these include ergot, pituitary extracts and quinine. Other substances normally used in obstetrics, particularly prostaglandins, are also used to induce abortions and are potentially more potent. However, in early pregnancy the uterus is not primed to respond to these drugs. Another group of chemicals is the strong purgatives such as colocynth, croton oil or jalap, which simply cause general debility to the woman, but they are highly unlikely to cause an abortion.

Instrumentation is commonly practised, involving a wide variety of devices from surgical probes and bougies to the crudest implements made of metal or wood, as well as bicycle spokes, metal coat-hangers or even twigs from trees. The dangers of instrumentation are perforation and infection. Medical or paramedical abortionists may have an adequate knowledge of the anatomy of the female genital tract and of the need for the instruments to be clean and preferably sterile, and so the dangers are less than with the same acts performed by many lay people who have no idea of the structure of the genital tract or of the need for cleanliness.

Instruments may be forced through the vaginal walls, especially the posterior fornix, or through the walls of the cervix or uterus. The fundus may be perforated and the instrument pushed up into the intestines or even the liver. All of these injuries can cause rapid death from haemorrhage or shock or delayed death from haemorrhage, shock and infection. The Higginson syringe (widely sold as a method of giving an enema) is still used as a means of inducing an abortion, despite its continued association with fatal air embolism.

Local interference other than instrumentation may take the form of chemicals applied to the cervix or interior of the uterus. Potassium permanganate crystals applied to the upper vagina and cervix have caused chemical burns and death from absorption of permanganate. Chemical mixtures ('Utus Paste' or 'Interruptin') were once used to induce therapeutic abortions by acting as endometrial irritants.

General violence in an attempt to induce a 'spontaneous' abortion may still be encountered on rare occasions. This may involve widespread injury from the infliction of multiple injuries or from a fall down stairs or from a height, or there may be more localized direct blunt injury (often punching or kicking) to the abdominal wall. These injures may be self-inflicted or they may be inflicted by the husband, the father or some other 'helper'. The more diffuse injuries will be very difficult to distinguish from an assault that may possibly have been occasioned by the announcement of the pregnancy.

Other methods that are thought to be capable of inducing a 'spontaneous' abortion include the taking of very hot baths, ingestion of large quantities of alcohol, vaginal douches with many substances, and violent exercise such as skipping, jumping and even riding horses or bicycles over rough ground. However, fetuses are generally very persistent and these methods very seldom work. Indeed, pregnant women who die as a result of trauma (for instance road traffic accidents) usually have no evidence of dislodgement of the pregnancy.

Syringe aspiration is a method used by both legal and criminal abortionists. A large syringe with an attached plastic cannula is pushed through the cervix, suction is applied, which ruptures the early gestational sac and leads to aspiration or later expulsion of the contents.

The dangerous or fatal effects of illegal abortion consist of:

- haemorrhage from local genital trauma during clumsy instrumental interference;

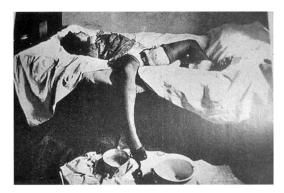

Figure 19.1 A photograph of only historic interest in the UK. This woman had died of air embolism after attempting to induce an abortion with a Higginson syringe, which can be seen below her right foot.

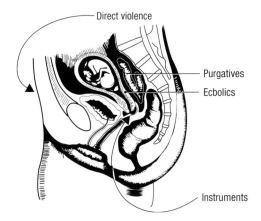

Figure 19.2 Diagram of a midline section of the female pelvic organs to illustrate the various sites of action of methods designed to induce an abortion.

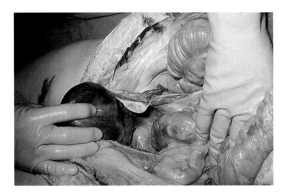

Figure 19.3 Autopsy appearance of a septic uterus following an illegal abortion.

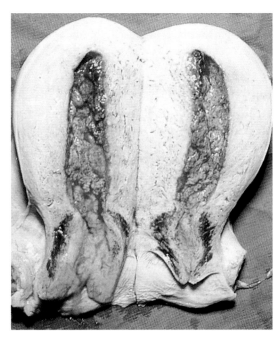

Figure 19.4 Septic endometritis after an illegal abortion. The haemorrhagic tracks in the cervix show where the instrument has pierced the cervical canal.

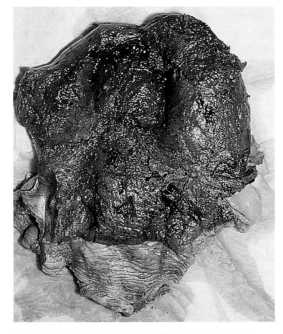

Figure 19.5 *Clostridium perfringens* infection ('gas gangrene') following an illegal abortion.

- sepsis due to the use of non-sterile instruments or methods and the lack of antibiotic prophylaxis;
- 'shock', which may be associated with haemorrhage or perforation of the vagina, uterus or adjacent organs; it may also be an immediate and sometimes fatal response to the dilatation of the cervix of an unanaesthetized woman;
- air embolism, which may occur during any form of instrumentation within the uterus, although injection of fluid into the uterus (with a Higginson syringe) is a common cause;
- later systemic complications, which include: thrombosis of the leg and pelvic veins with the subsequent risk of fatal pulmonary embolism; infection, which brings the risk of septicaemia and the associated complications of disseminated intravascular coagulation; hepatic and renal failure etc; and
- sterility, which is a very common complication of these highly dangerous procedures.

Legal termination of pregnancy

Many countries now have legal provisions for the medical termination of pregnancy. This is often called 'therapeutic abortion', which is not exactly synonymous with 'medical termination' because in some countries a woman has the right to have an 'abortion on demand' without having to satisfy any medical preconditions; such an operation can hardly be called 'therapeutic'.

Most countries, including Britain, require that some medical condition be proved before the abortion is sanctioned, though the scope and strictness of such proof vary widely.

The Hippocratic Oath totally banned the involvement of doctors in abortions, a view that was confirmed by the World Medical Association Declaration of Geneva in 1948. This view was modified by the same association 22 years later in 1970, when the Declaration of Oslo was approved, which accepted that doctors could participate in abortions but only where this was sanctioned by the laws of their own country.

The Roman Catholic and Islamic religions are fundamentally opposed to any termination of pregnancy, although most religious codes would not prohibit the truly therapeutic termination of a pregnancy in a woman who was likely to die if the pregnancy proceeded to full term. The Infant Life Preservation Act of 1929 gave limited protection to a doctor who performed an abortion 'for the purpose only of preserving the life of the mother', provided that the operation was performed in good faith.

The wide variation in the laws and regulations that relate to abortions from country to country means that it is impossible to give an account here of the different legal provisions for termination of pregnancy around the world. These laws and regulations are changing all the time, some countries becoming more liberal while others become more restrictive. One of the best-known pieces of legislation that allows for therapeutic abortion on medical grounds was the Abortion Act of 1967, which relates to England, Wales and Scotland but not to Northern Ireland. This Abortion Act was modified in 1990 by the Human Fertilization and Embryology Act. The fundamental rules governing the provision of staff and premises for abortions and the four circumstances that allow for a decision to be taken to perform a therapeutic abortion are set out below.

RULES

- The termination must be performed by a registered medical practitioner.
- It must be carried out in a Health Service hospital or a place specifically registered for the purpose.
- Two registered medical practitioners must examine the woman (not necessarily together) and certify that grounds for termination exist. Neither of these doctors needs to be the doctor who actually performs the operation.
- The termination must be notified to medical officers of the appropriate government department.

CIRCUMSTANCES

- The pregnancy must not exceed its twenty-fourth week and that the continuance of pregnancy would involve risk, greater than if the pregnancy were terminated, of injury to the physical or mental health of the pregnant woman or any existing children of her family; **or**
- The termination is necessary to prevent grave permanent injury to the physical or mental health of the pregnant woman; **or**
- The continuance of the pregnancy would involve risk to the life of the pregnant woman, greater than if the pregnancy were terminated; **or**

- There is a substantial risk that if the child were born, it would suffer from such physical or mental abnormalities as to be seriously handicapped.

In an emergency, to save the life of or to prevent 'grave permanent injury to the physical or mental health of the pregnant woman', a termination may be carried out anywhere on the certification of only one medical practitioner.

Consent to termination of pregnancy

The rules for consent to a termination of pregnancy are no different from those applicable to any other medical or surgical procedure. In most Western countries (where therapeutic abortion is lawful), the only consent that is required for termination of pregnancy is from the woman herself, provided she is competent to make that decision. The consent of a husband or permanent partner (if he accompanies the woman) may be obtained as good clinical practice; however, the woman's wishes are paramount and a husband's or partner's objections are not relevant in English law. It is possible that when the grounds for the abortion are the health of the children of the existing family, the views of the husband may be relevant and may influence the decision of the two certifying doctors.

The consent or otherwise of a more casual 'boyfriend' or even the putative father of the child is not relevant and although several attempts have been made through the courts to establish the right of the putative father to object to an abortion of 'his' child, none has yet succeeded.

Any competent young girl may seek medial advice and may consent on her own to an abortion, although for girls under 16 the doctor should seek to encourage them to discuss the matter with their parents or carers. This principle was established in 1985 by a ruling from the House of Lords in the Gillick case. The key question is the competence of the girl and if, in the opinion of the doctor who will perform the abortion, she is capable of understanding the details, implications and possible consequences of the abortion, she can legally consent. There are two exceptions, one absolute and one partial. The absolute exception is a girl who is a ward of court, in which case only the court can give consent; the partial exception is a girl who is legally in the care of the local authority, in which case the British Medical Association advises that it would be prudent for the consent of her carers to be obtained.

Conversely, a girl of any fertile age, even under 16, certainly cannot be made to have an abortion on the wishes of her parents or anyone else if she herself does not agree.

Chapter twenty

Deaths and Injury in Infancy

The results and effects of disease and trauma are, in general terms, similar in all victims, but there are some special features of injuries to infants and children that require consideration. It is important to remember that babies and children are not just small adults and they have their own unique problems, such as still-birth and sudden infant death syndrome, which have important medico-legal aspects. They are also particularly dependent and hence vulnerable to abuse, both physical and sexual.

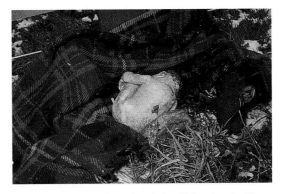

Figure 20.1 The body of a newborn baby with the placenta still attached was left in a blanket by the side of a country road. At autopsy, no evidence of a separate existence could be proved.

STILLBIRTHS

A significant number of pregnancies that continue into the third trimester fail to deliver a live child and result in a stillbirth. The definitions of a stillbirth vary from country to country, but the British definition, which dates from 1990 and takes into account the advances in resuscitation and care of premature infants, is perhaps typical: the child must be of more than 24 weeks' gestational age and, after being completely expelled from the mother, did not breathe or show any signs of life. These 'signs of life', in addition to respiration and heart beat, are taken to mean movement, crying or pulsation of the umbilical cord.

If death has occurred more than a couple of days before birth, the fetus is commonly macerated due to the effects of early decomposition combined with exposure to fluid. The infant is discoloured, usually a pinkish-brown or red, with extensive desquamation of the skin; the tissues have a soft, slimy translucence and there may be partial collapse of the head with over-riding of the skull plates. The appearance of the child is quite different from that seen in an infant who has died following a live birth and then begun to putrefy. Because many, if not most, of these deaths occur after the onset of labour and during the process of birth itself, no evidence of decomposition will be present.

In English law, a child does not have a 'separate existence' (and thus does not become a legal person, capable of acquiring legal rights of inheritance, title etc.) until he or she is completely free from the mother's body, though the cord and placenta may still be within the mother. The Infant Life Preservation Act (1929) made it an offence to destroy a baby during birth; however, an exception was made in the Act for doctors acting 'in good faith' who, to save the life of the mother, have to destroy a baby that becomes impacted in the pelvis during birth.

As babies who are stillborn have never 'lived' in the legal sense, they cannot 'die' and so a death certificate cannot be issued. In Britain, a special 'stillbirth certificate' may be completed either by a doctor or a midwife if either was present at the birth or by either one of them if they have examined the body of the child after birth.

The causes of stillbirth are varied and may be undeterminable, even after a full autopsy. Indeed, it may be impossible to determine on the pathological features alone if the death occurred before, during or after birth. Recognized conditions leading to intrauterine or perimortem death include prematurity, fetal hypoxia, placental insufficiency, intra-uterine infections (viral, bacterial or fungal), congenital defects (especially in the cardiovascular or nervous system) and birth trauma.

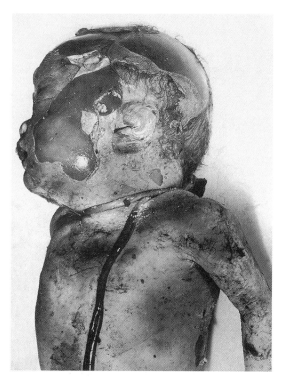

Figure 20.2 A newborn infant showing marked maceration due to an intrauterine death. The cord around the neck is significant, but a full autopsy is required to establish the cause of death.

INFANTICIDE

The term infanticide has a very specific meaning in the many countries that have introduced legislation designed to circumvent the criminal charge of murder when a mother kills her child during its first year of life. The Infanticide Act of England and Wales states that:

> Where a woman by a wilful act of omission or commission causes the death of her child being under the age of twelve months but at the time the balance of her mind was disturbed by the effects of childbirth or lactation she may be dealt with as if she had committed manslaughter.

Because manslaughter is a less serious charge than murder and does not result in the mandatory penalty of life imprisonment that is attached to murder, a verdict of infanticide allows the court to make an appropriate sentence for the mother, which is more likely to be probation and psychiatric supervision than custody. The Infanticide Act recognizes the special nature of infanticide and the particular effects pregnancy and lactation may have upon the woman.

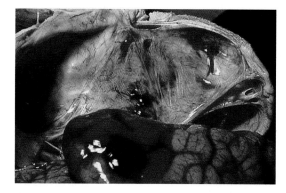

Figure 20.3 Examination of the brain of a newborn infant shows haemorrhage over the temporal lobe due to an unattended and precipitate birth.

In English law, there is a presumption that all dead babies are stillborn and so the onus is on the prosecution, and hence the pathologist, to prove that the child was born alive and had a separate existence. In order to do this, it must be shown that the infant breathed or showed other signs of life, such as movement or pulsation of the umbilical cord, after having been completely expelled from the mother.

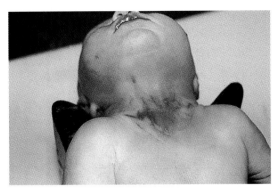

Figure 20.4 Abrasion of the neck of a baby. These marks were said to have been caused by traction of the neck of the baby by the mother during self-delivery. Similar marks could be caused by strangulation.

In the absence of eyewitness accounts, pathologists can make no comment about the viability or otherwise of a baby at the moment of complete expulsion from the mother, and one way that they may be able to comment on the possibility of separate existence is if they can establish that the child had breathed. However, establishing that breathing had taken place is still not absolute evidence of a 'separate existence', as a baby in a vertex delivery can breathe after the head and thorax have been delivered but before delivery of the lower body.

The 'flotation test', which used to be the definitive test for breathing, and hence separate existence, and which was depended upon for many centuries, is now considered to be unreliable – although it still appears in some textbooks. All that can be said with regard to flotation of the lungs is that if a lung or piece of lung sinks in water, the baby had not breathed sufficiently to expand that lung and so the child may have been stillborn. The converse is definitely not true, as the lungs of babies who are proven to have been stillborn sometimes float. This test is useless in differentiating between live-born and stillborn infants and should no longer be used.

Some textbooks recommend sets of highly complicated procedures at autopsy in an attempt to resolve this problem, but all of these tests are far too unreliable and unpredictable and although they might allow for medical speculation and discussion, they do not allow the pathologist to say, in court, under oath and beyond all reasonable doubt, that a child has or has not breathed.

To complicate matters further, many dead newborn babies are hidden and may not be discovered

until decomposition has begun, which precludes any reliable assessment of the state of expansion of the lungs. Even in fresh bodies, the problems are immense and any attempt at mouth-to-mouth resuscitation or even chest compression will prevent any reliable opinion being given on the possibility of spontaneous breathing.

On the other hand, if there is milk in the stomach or if the stump of the umbilical cord is shrivelled or shows an inflammatory ring of impending separation, the child must have lived for some time after birth.

Establishing the identity of the infant and the identity of the mother is often a matter of great difficulty, as these babies are often found hidden or abandoned. When the baby is found in the home, there is seldom any dispute about who the mother is. Commonly, it is a teenage girl, usually unmarried and sometimes even unaware that she was pregnant until the birth occurred.

In those cases where the mother is traced, further legal action depends on whether the pathologist can definitely decide if the baby was born alive or was stillborn. If live-born, no charge of infanticide can be brought in English law unless a wilful act of omission or commission can be proved to have caused the death. Omission means the deliberate failure to provide the normal care at birth such as tying and cutting the cord, clearing the air passages of mucus and keeping the baby warm and fed. The wilful or deliberate withholding of these acts, as opposed to the ignorance and inexperience of a frightened teenage girl, is hard to establish. Acts of commission are more straightforward for the doctor to demonstrate as they include head injuries, stabbing, drowning, strangulation etc.

The maturity of the infant is rarely an issue as most infants found dead after birth are at or near full term of 38–40 weeks. The legal age of maturity in Britain is now 24 weeks, though medical advances have allowed fetuses of only 20 weeks' or less gestation to survive in specialist neonatal units. In infanticide, the maturity is not legally material as it is the deliberate killing of any baby that has attained a separate existence, and this does not depend directly upon the gestational age.

THE ESTIMATION OF MATURITY OF A NEWBORN BABY OR FETUS

It may be necessary to estimate the length of gestation from the body of a baby or fetus in relation to an abortion, stillbirth or alleged infanticide. Two very rough 'rule of thumb' formulae for estimating maturity are:

1 up to the twentieth week, the length of the fetus in centimetres is the square of the age in months (Haase's rule);
2 after the twentieth week, the length of the fetus in centimetres equals five times the age in months.

There is considerable variation in any of the measured parameters due to sex, race, nutrition and individual variation, but it is possible to form a reasonable estimate of the maturity of a fetus by using the brief notes that follow.

4 weeks	1.25 cm, showing limb buds, enveloped in villous chorion.
12 weeks	9 cm long, nails formed on digits, placenta well formed, lanugo all over body.
20 weeks	18–25 cm, weight 350–450 g, hair on head.
24 weeks	30 cm crown–heel, vernix on skin.
28 weeks	35 cm crown–heel, 25 cm crown–rump, weight 900–1400 g.
32 weeks	40 cm crown–heel, weight 1500–2000 g.
36 weeks	45 cm crown–heel, weight 2200 g.
40 weeks (full term)	48–52 cm crown–heel, 28–32 cm crown–rump, 33–38 cm head circumference, lanugo now absent or present only over shoulders, head hair up to 2–3 cm long, testes palpable in scrotum/vulval labia close vaginal opening, dark meconium in large intestine.

Development can also be assessed using the ossification centres and the histological appearances of the

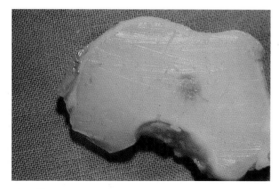

Figure 20.5 Cross-section of the lower end of the femur showing the ossification centre.

major organs. Specialist anthropological and paediatric textbooks should be consulted for further details of any of these methods.

SUDDEN INFANT DEATH SYNDROME

Sudden infant death syndrome (SIDS) is also known as 'cot death' or 'crib death' and in westernized countries now has an incidence of approximately 0.6 per 1000 live births, which is a considerable reduction from the early 1990s when the incidence was between 1.5 and 2 per 1000 live births. The decline in SIDS deaths began in 1991 and has accelerated since the introduction in 1994 of the worldwide 'Back to Sleep' campaign, which encouraged mothers to place babies on their back to sleep rather than face down or on their side. Publicity campaigns have also advised mothers to refrain from smoking during pregnancy or near to their babies after birth and to avoid overheating babies by wrapping them up too closely. However, despite this significant decline, SIDS still forms the most common cause of death in the post-perinatal period in countries with a relatively low infant mortality rate.

A definition of SIDS may be stated as 'the sudden death of an infant which is unexpected by history and by examination of the scene and in whom a thorough autopsy fails to reveal an adequate cause of death'. The following are the main features of the syndrome.

- The accepted age range is between 2 weeks and 2 years, but most deaths takes place between 1 and 7 months, with a peak at 2–3 months.
- There is little sex difference, although there is a slight preponderance of males similar to that seen in many types of death.
- The incidence is markedly greater in multiple births, whether identical or not. This can be partly explained by the greater incidence of premature and low birth-weight infants in multiple births.
- There is a marked seasonal variation in temperate zones: SIDS is far more common in the colder and wetter months, in both the Northern and Southern hemispheres.
- There are apparent social, racial and ethnic differences, but these are explained by fundamental underlying socio-economic factors, which show that there is a higher incidence in any disadvantaged families such as those with poor housing, lower

occupational status, one-parent families etc. However, no class, race or creed is exempt from these devastating deaths.

The essence of SIDS is that the deaths are unexpected and autopsy reveals no adequate cause of death. The history is usually typical: a perfectly well child – or one with only trivial symptoms – is put in the sleeping place at night only to be found dead in the morning. At autopsy, nothing specific is found in the true SIDS death, although in about 70 per cent of cases the autopsy reveals intrathoracic petechiae on the pleura, epicardium and thymus, which formerly gave rise to the misapprehension that SIDS was due to mechanical suffocation. These are now believed to be agonal phenomena and not a cause of death.

The true aetiology of SIDS is unknown, but it is likely that there are many different causes, often multifactorial, which act via a final common pathway of cardiorespiratory failure. Theories about possible 'causes' of SIDS abound and include allergy to cows' milk or house-mites, botulism, prolonged sleep apnoea, spinal haemorrhages, deficiencies of liver enzymes, selenium or vitamin E, various metabolic defects, vaccinations, hyperthermia, hypothermia, carbon monoxide or dioxide poisoning, viral bronchiolitis, muscle hypotonia, and many others. As yet, none of these has been substantiated.

One persistent claim is for a possible role of deliberate mechanical suffocation by the wilful action of a parent. Speculation that up to 10 per cent of SIDS are caused in this way is difficult to refute but has never been substantiated by confessions, statistics or research.

The doctor must certainly be vigilant in any infant death, but the dangers of reinforcing the inevitable guilt in the great majority of innocent parents must be weighed against the chance of detecting a deliberate suffocation. The doctor's main concern in the management of SIDS is to support the family by explanations and to make sure that the counselling services established in many Western countries are made available to the parents.

CHILD ABUSE

Child abuse is a major social problem, which involves many medical specialties including paediatricians, general practitioners, psychiatrists and forensic practitioners. Child abuse is a generic term that covers both the physical and sexual abuse of children.

Child physical abuse

The syndrome of physical abuse was noticed in the middle of the twentieth century by doctors such as Caffey, who was a radiologist and who described limb fractures and subdural haemorrhages in infants that he first thought were due to a new disease. Subsequently, this combination of injuries was shown to be due to ill-treatment by the carers. In fact, Caffey and his co-workers had only rediscovered a syndrome, as similar features had been described by Tardieu in Paris during the middle of the nineteenth century.

Following the description by Caffey and others of this syndrome – variously called 'baby battering' or 'non-accidental injury' – there was a very significant increase in the frequency with which it was diagnosed and it is not entirely clear if this increase was due simply to increased awareness of the syndrome leading to increased reporting or whether it was due to a true increase in the incidence of abuse. It is most likely that there is truth in both of those statements. All types of child abuse are more frequently reported in the more advanced, industrialized countries, but there is no doubt that it is a global problem.

The threshold between actions that are accepted as legitimate physical punishment of a child by a parent, carer or other authority figure (school teacher etc.) varies with time, geography and culture. What was approved in the Victorian era as 'beneficial chastisement' would now almost certainly be condemned as cruelty, and some countries have gone so far as to prohibit all forms of physical chastisement of children by anyone, including their parents.

EPIDEMIOLOGY

The physically abused child can be of either sex and of any age. Fatalities are more common in children under the age of 2 years. Sexually abused children tend to be slightly older, although this may reflect the problems in perceiving and reporting sexual abuse in very young children. The upper age limit is very difficult to define: physical abuse is more likely to stop at a younger age, whereas sexual abuse commonly continues into the teens and even older. In developed societies, there is no clear distinction in incidence between the different social strata, but there may be a slight preponderance in the families of skilled manual workers.

GENERAL FEATURES

There are four general features that should make doctors suspicious that they are dealing with injuries that are the result of physical child abuse and not from a childhood accident:

1 if the child has suffered from repeated injuries;
2 if there is a delay in seeking medical assistance by the carers;
3 if the child has been taken to different hospitals or doctors for treatment of the different injuries; or
4 if the explanation(s) given by the carer(s) does not correlate with the type or the extent of the injuries that are present on the child.

Any child suspected of being a victim of physical child abuse should be fully examined by an experienced practitioner and every injury, old or recent, should be carefully recorded on a diagram, in the written notes and, if possible, by photography. All of the skin of the child should be examined for injuries, although this does not mean that the child has to be examined naked because this may cause great distress to some children.

INJURIES

Bruising

All children will sustain injuries that result in bruising on many occasions while they are growing up. These injuries are particularly common when children begin to mobilize and later when they begin to play and to explore their environment. The type and extent of injury that may reasonably be found on a child will vary with their age and the environment in which they are living. One would not expect a toddler to have multiple bruises of varying ages on his lower legs, whereas that pattern of injury would be acceptable (indeed, it might be almost expected) in an enthusiastic 10-year-old footballer.

The features of bruises that are important can be summed up as site, age and multiplicity. Bruising of the arms and legs, especially around the upper arms, forearms, wrists, ankles and knees, may be evidence of

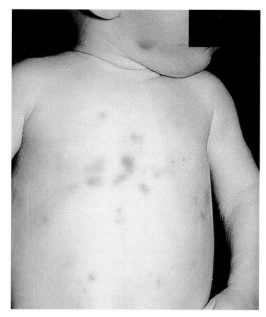

Figure 20.6 Fingertip bruises on the chest and abdomen of a child who died in the care of its mother's boyfriend. Autopsy revealed a ruptured liver.

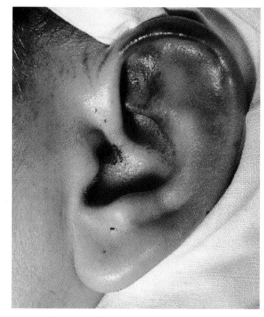

Figure 20.7 Bruising of the ear of a small child. X-rays revealed multiple rib fractures suggestive of child abuse.

gripping by an adult. Bruises on the face, ears, lips, neck, lateral thorax, anterior abdomen, buttocks and thighs are very suspicious, as these sites are less likely to be injured in childhood falls.

The age of an injury cannot be reliably determined (see Chapter 9) from the colour of the bruise alone. However, areas of bruising on the same part of the body that show different colours are a strong indication that the injuries are of different ages, and multiple injuries inflicted over a period of time are highly suspicious of physical abuse.

The explanation given by the carers of how all of the injuries present on the child were caused must be noted with great care for two reasons: firstly, so that the doctor understands exactly what happened, allowing for a good interpretation of the injuries; and secondly, so that any changes in the explanation given by the carers over time or to different individuals can be compared.

Skeletal injury

Fractures, displaced epiphyses and other evidence of skeletal trauma are highly suggestive of physical child abuse. X-rays of the living child should be used sparingly, but suspected physical child abuse is one condition for which a full skeletal survey is justified. These considerations of radiation risk do not affect the pathologist, who should always examine the x-rays of a full skeletal survey before commencing an examination in suspected physical child abuse. It is also important to consider physical abuse when examining any x-ray of a child, even when that diagnosis is not under immediate consideration. If there is any doubt about features seen on an x-ray of a child, the films must be reviewed by a paediatric radiologist.

Recent fractures, especially of the skull, ribs and limbs, are of particular significance, but evidence of previous fractures is also vital in confirming long-term abuse. Old fractures and trauma can be indicated by callus formation, subperiosteal calcification in old haematomas, slipped epiphyses, metaphyseal damage etc. The classical radiological picture of a child who has been physically abused shows a combination of recent and old fractures with areas of callus formation.

Rib fractures are rarely accidental in children. They may occasionally be associated with birth trauma, but in general they are a feature of the application of substantial force. One particular pattern that may be seen on x-ray or at autopsy comprises areas of callus on the posterior ribs, often lying in a line adjacent to the vertebrae, and giving a 'string-of-beads' appearance. This pattern is interpreted as indicating an episode or episodes of forceful squeezing of the chest by adult hands. The possibility that even amateur or inexperienced and over-enthusiastic cardiopulmonary resuscitation can cause multiple rib fractures is remote, given the tremendously flexible nature of a baby's or young infant's ribs.

A skull fracture is always a marker of significant trauma to the head, and skull fractures are common in fatal cases of physical child abuse, but they are not necessarily accompanied by brain damage. They often comprise a linear split across the temporal or parietal bones, which may sometimes cross the sagittal suture. Less often, fractures of the occipital or frontal bones are present and basal fractures are uncommon.

Research in Germany has demonstrated that skull fractures in children can be caused by passive falls from only 80 cm onto carpeted floors. For comparison, the seat of a 'standard' settee or chair is about 40 cm from the floor, the mattress of a 'standard' bed about 60 cm from the floor, and a 'standard' tabletop is about 70 cm from the floor. These figures would suggest that, unless the furniture was unusually high, or some other factors have to be considered, falls from furniture onto the floor are unlikely to be the cause of a skull fracture in a child.

Head injuries

Head injuries are the most frequent cause of death in child abuse, and even when they are non-fatal, they may result in severe and permanent neurological disability. Head injuries may be caused in one of two ways: direct trauma to the head and shaking (shaken baby syndrome). Subdural haemorrhages, cerebral trauma and axonal damage can be caused by both of these mechanisms, whereas skull fractures can only be caused by direct trauma. Discussion continues about the more likely cause of the intracranial injuries in children who have no evidence of direct trauma to the head. Many paediatricians favour shaking as a mechanism and, although many pathologists would accept this, they are also aware that significant direct trauma to the head – especially from a broad object such as a hand – may not leave any mark of that impact.

Perhaps the important factors here are not so much the exact mechanism of delivery of the energy to the head of the child, but how much energy is delivered and how quickly. Some research suggests that the forces delivered to the head from a 'substantial' blow can be many times greater than those delivered by shaking, but if the lesser forces of shaking are more than sufficient to cause intercranial injury, this research is of little value in understanding the mechanism of that injury. Whether from direct blows or from shaking, it is clear that if sufficient force is applied to the head of a child, the ultimate effects are brain injury and that injury carries with it a substantial risk of disability or death.

Ocular injuries

The eyes can often provide good evidence of physical abuse, as up to 70 per cent of physically abused infants have eye lesions, including retinal haemorrhages, vitreous haemorrhage, dislocated lens or detached retina. Suspected victims of child abuse should be seen by a doctor who is competent in ophthalmoscopic examination. Examination of the eyes should always be part of a post-mortem examination in fatal cases of suspected child abuse.

Oral injuries

The lips may be bruised or abraded by blows to the face and, if the child is old enough to have teeth, the inner side of the lips may be bruised or lacerated by contact with the tooth edges. A characteristic lesion of physical child abuse is a torn frenulum inside the lip; this can be damaged either by a tangential blow across the mouth or by an object, sometimes a feeding bottle, being rammed forcibly into the mouth between lip and gum.

Visceral injuries

Visceral injuries are the second most frequent cause of death and it is the organs of the abdomen – the intestine, mesentery and liver – that are most commonly injured. The anterior abdominal wall of a child offers little or no protection against direct trauma from fist or foot, and blows from the front can trap the duodenum, the jejunum or the mesentery between the compressed abdominal wall and the anvil of the lumbar spine. This compression crushes the tissues and may even result in transection of the bowel, with the obvious consequences of peritonitis and shock. Crushing or rupturing of the mesentery may lead to bruising or to frank intraperitoneal bleeding.

The liver is relatively large in a child and protrudes below the rib cage, and it can be ruptured by direct blows to the abdomen. However, the spleen is rarely damaged in physical child abuse due to its relatively sheltered position.

Other injuries

Other injuries in physical child abuse include burns and bites. Burns can be caused in many ways: from the application of heated metal objects or cigarettes to the hands, legs, buttocks or torso or to scalding due to immersion in hot water or from splashing from hot water that is thrown (see Chapter 15). Cigarette burns have a typical appearance: they are commonly circular and, when fresh, are pink or red in colour and have an excavated appearance; ash may be see at the base of the burn crater. When healing, they tend to be silvery in the centre with a narrow red rim. A single scar left by a cigarette burn is non-specific, but multiple round scars on the body in association with a history of these burns can be diagnostic.

Bites also occur in child abuse and they are commonly multiple. They must be differentiated from bites from siblings, other children or even domestic pets. Swabs from a fresh bite should be taken as soon as possible, as they may recover saliva, which can be subjected to DNA analysis. The advice of a dentist, preferably a forensic odontologist, should also be sought as soon as possible, as the shape of the bite can be matched (by measurement, photography or latex casts) to the dentition of a suspected assailant.

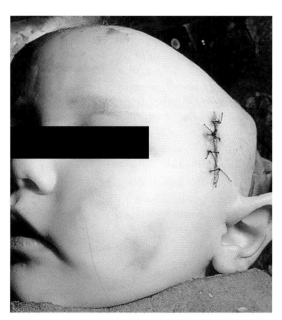

Figure 20.8 An adult bite mark on the face of an abused child. An operation site for draining the fatal subdural haemorrhage can be seen.

Genuine accidents to children are far more frequent than acts of child physical abuse. However, it can be extremely difficult to distinguish between them. Any doctor who examines children must always bear in mind the possibility of physical child abuse – even in the well-spoken, middle-class family – and although it is vital that innocent parents are not unjustly accused of ill-treating their children, it is equally important that abuse is recognized, as the next time the child, or a sibling, presents for treatment may be when he is fatally injured or dead.

Child sexual abuse

The problem of the sexual abuse and exploitation of children is global and thousands of children are sexually abused every day around the world. Sexual abuse has come to prominence more recently than physical abuse, although sexual contact between adults and children has been recorded in many situations and many countries for centuries. The modern definition of child sexual abuse may be expressed as 'the involvement of dependent, developmentally immature children and adolescents in sexual activities they do not truly comprehend, to which they are unable to give informed consent or which violate social taboos or family roles'.

The diagnosis and management of child sexual abuse are multidisciplinary, involving not only doctors but also social agencies and sometimes law enforcement agencies. On the medical side, there needs to be a partnership between paediatricians and forensic medical examiners (police surgeons), although in general terms the physical findings on medical examination may be minimal or absent, especially if the abuse is not reported for weeks, months or even years after the actual events, and may form only a very small part of the diagnosis.

Great care needs to be exercised in the examination of the suspected victims of sexual abuse, and specialist doctors are now available throughout the UK. If no specialist doctors are available and the opinions of both a paediatrician and a forensic practitioner are needed, arrangements must be made for a joint examination so that the search for physical signs and the retention of samples for forensic tests can be done together. When more than 72 hours have passed since intercourse, the chances of recovering sperm from the vagina are too low to make the taking of high vaginal swabs justified, but swabs of the introitus and examination of underwear should be considered.

In general terms, much of the examination routine is similar to that recommended in sexual offences against older age groups: history-taking, consent, confidentiality, good examination facilities and the need for a general examination before any perineal examination are all essential, but uppermost in the mind of the doctor must be the concern that any further psychological trauma to the child is avoided.

The possibility of sexually transmitted diseases being present must always be borne in mind. This has both forensic and therapeutic aspects for the examining doctor, because they may provide a positive link to a perpetrator while also needing urgent treatment.

The difficulties of getting accurate evidence or a witness statement from a very immature witness and placing it before a court have led to the use of video-recorded interviews and examinations including the use of dolls to indicate parts of the body. These interviews must be performed by specially trained individuals – usually police officers or social workers.

No doctor should voluntarily commence an examination of a child who might have been sexually abused without having had paediatric and forensic training, because it is the appreciation of the wide range of normal appearances of the genitalia and anus that is the key-stone of a reliable opinion, and there is great concern that unless the doctor has had this specialist training, the value of his or her opinion to a court may be reduced. Extensive, clear notes must, of course, be taken, with diagrams to support the text.

Digital examination of the vagina in a pre-pubertal child is rarely indicated and may need to be performed under general anaesthesia if thought to be absolutely essential.

Chapter twenty-one

Neglect, Starvation and Abuse of Human Rights

PHYSICAL ABUSE OF HUMAN RIGHTS: TORTURE

In an increasingly violent and divided world, abuses of human rights, both physical and psychological, are more common. The term 'ethnic cleansing' has been added to the vocabulary, and concentration camps, mass rape and murder and the torture of men, women and children have again been seen in Europe in the last decade. Regrettably, about one-third of the member states of the United Nations have been involved in these abhorrent activities during the past few decades, even though they are all signatories to declarations outlawing such practices.

The 1975 Tokyo Declaration of the World Medical Association on 'Torture and other cruel and degrading treatment or punishment' specifically forbids the involvement of medical practitioners in the administration of torture, and this view is strongly reinforced by the British Medical Association in its report on 'The Medical Profession and Human Rights: handbook for a changing agenda'.

Forensic practitioners have a crucial primary role to play in the impartial examination of individuals who reach asylum and claim refugee status. In this situation, the authorities of the host country often require definite forensic evidence that will support a claim of torture in order to verify the request for asylum based on physical abuse.

If the injuries are fresh, their documentation and interpretation will generally follow the standard route and practices of the examination of a victim of a violent physical assault. However, one of the major problems faced by the doctor is the long interval, often of months or even years, that will commonly have elapsed between the infliction of the injuries and the date of examination. This delay in examination is often inevitable due to periods of imprisonment and delays while the victim manages to escape to a country of sanctuary. During this time, the normal healing processes will occur and many acute injuries will disappear completely, while others will remain as scars. It requires very careful examination combined with experience of either similar cases or of forensic medicine to detect and interpret such old lesions.

Features of physical abuse

The ways of deliberately harming victims are limited only by the ingenuity of the torturers, and the forensic evidence left upon the body of the victim will reflect the methods used. Blunt trauma, sharp trauma, application of heat or electricity, asphyxia and suspension are all commonly encountered.

Beating with a variety of objects is the most common form of abuse and will result in the usual triad of signs associated with that type of trauma: bruising,

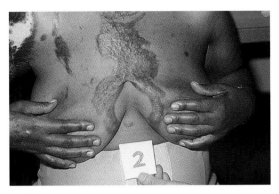

Figure 21.1 This woman was tied to a chair beneath a burning car tyre. The dripping burning rubber caused these injuries.

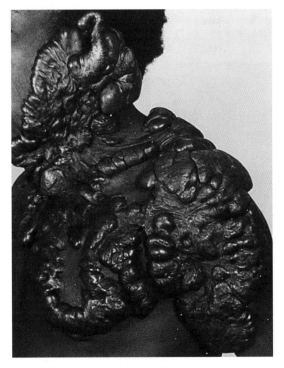

Figure 21.2 Extreme keloid scarring following burns inflicted by an electric hot plate and burning rags.

abrasion and laceration. Particular weapons or objects may leave particular patterns on the skin, for example a blow from a rod or thong will commonly result in parallel tramline bruises (see Chapter 9). Healing of these bruises and abrasions will generally be complete and leave no residual signs, although in some dark-skinned victims there is sometimes a linear increase in pigmentation that may provide permanent evidence. Where the skin is lacerated, the scar left may provide clear evidence of the site of the injury. Susceptible individuals may develop keloid scarring.

The sites of injury are very variable; blows to the head, back, buttocks, perineum and soles of the feet ('falanga') are favourite places for beating. Falanga consists of the soles of the feet being beaten with a thin rod or cane and, because of the thick skin and dense fascia at this site, permanent signs of injury are slight even though deep tenderness may be long-lasting after the initial pain and swelling have subsided.

Cutting and piercing injuries are common features of torture; knives, bayonets, glass fragments, needles or any object with a cutting edge or a point may be used on any part of the body. The injuries may be incised wounds, stab wounds or a combination of the two. The resulting scar may reflect the type of injury caused.

Burns may be inflicted from anything that will either burn or can be heated: cigarette lighters, hot irons, electric heating rings, branding irons, cigarettes, ignited kerosene-soaked rags or molten rubber. Acutely, the burns show the usual features, but if healing has occurred, the residual lesions will depend upon the site and severity of the burns.

Burns can also be caused by both acid and caustic materials, the favourite being sulphuric acid in the form of 'battery fluid'. These chemicals, if strong enough, will damage skin and eyes. Their fluid nature can often be confirmed by the presence of the typical trickle-marks of a corrosive fluid. Scarring will depend on the depth of the injury.

Electrical torture is excruciatingly painful and is often used because it leaves little permanent signs. The shocks can be of any voltage, but are most commonly taken direct from the mains supply of 110 or 240 V. Higher voltages derived from a magneto or a motor ignition coil have also been used. The electrodes may be clipped to, or bare wires applied to, the skin, tongue, breasts, nipples, penis or vulva. With mains voltage, the risk of fatal electrocution is present but seems rare, perhaps because of the short duration of each shock. The points of contact may leave small scars but, in general, the residual effects of electricity are almost undetectable in the living. If death occurs during or soon after electrical torture, special histological examination of the sites of electrocution can be used to confirm the presence of recent electrical injuries.

Damage to the ears is frequent, especially from the 'telefono' technique in which hands are clapped violently against the side of the head. This action may rupture the eardrum and damage the inner ear.

Suffocation and partial drowning are also employed, the usual intention being to partially asphyxiate, rather than kill. Immersion in water and foul sewage is termed 'wet submarino' and may lead to pneumonias. 'Dry submarino' is partial asphyxia by holding a plastic bag over the head. These activities can sometimes be inadvertently fatal.

Suspension is a common form of torture, the limbs being roped to a ceiling beam while the body hangs free beneath. Musculoskeletal injuries are very likely to result from these acts and they may result in permanent joint damage. These injuries may require examination by an expert in orthopaedics for accurate interpretation.

In addition to the physical lesions, gross psychiatric damage is very commonly caused, which will require careful and prolonged therapy by experts. A number of groups exist to offer their expertise in the verification of injuries and the diagnosis and treatment of both physical and mental suffering in these unfortunate victims of political, ethnic, religious and racial intolerance.

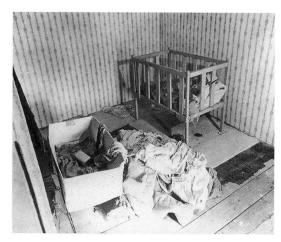

Figure 21.3 Scene of child neglect. The cardboard box was used as the cot for a baby in this unheated room. Frozen urine was found in the box.

NEGLECT AND STARVATION

Neglect and starvation are not identical but often go together; both can be self-inflicted or produced by others. They may be seen as a part of torture or deliberate abuse, but they may also be seen as separate entities with many other causes and associated factors.

Neglect seems to be more common in industrialized societies and is commonly associated with abuse in the old and very young, with mental abnormality (with or without alcohol or drug abuse) in the young and middle aged, and as a result of social isolation in the elderly, which is sometimes induced by senile dementia. Rarely is neglect due to sheer poverty.

When neglect is inflicted by others, children are the usual, but not exclusive, victims. Neglect is typified by excess dirt in the environment that the individual occupies. Commonly, that environment is also cold and poorly ventilated. Food, if available, will be of poor quality and of minimal quantity.

The poor nutrition of chronic starvation predisposes to infections and deficiency disorders, such as beri-beri and pellagra, so that skin conditions and internal disease become added to catabolic tissue loss caused by calorie deficiency. Emaciation is commonly the most obvious feature because, when the minimum calorie intake for an adult of about 1500 per day is not

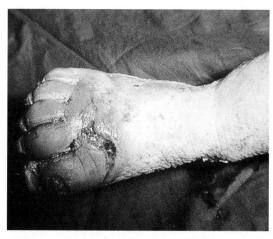

Figure 21.4 Frostbite of the foot in the child from Fig. 21.3. The actual cause of death was pneumonia. The body of the child had been disposed of by the parents down the farm well.

maintained over a period of time, body fat and then muscle mass will be lost. The calorie intake required by a child is disproportionately large and the exact figure will depend on age, size and level of activity.

When the body weight falls to less than 40 per cent of the original weight, there is danger of death, especially if the weight loss has been rapid. Complete deprivation of food in an adult is likely to cause death in about 50–60 days provided there is sufficient water for free intake. There are, however, great variations depending on the environment and the original state of fitness of the victim. On the other hand, life cannot last for more than about 10 days in a temperate climate without water.

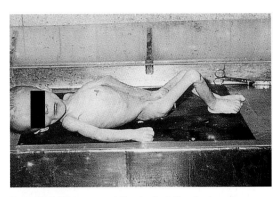

Figure 21.5 Extreme emaciation due to deliberate starvation, showing the scaphoid abdomen, shrunken limbs and 'Hippocratic facies' of dehydration and wasting.

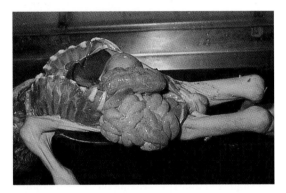

Figure 21.6 The abdominal contents of the child in Fig. 21.5. The bowel is empty apart from gas.

Two main types of starvation are described: the 'wet' and the 'dry'. The former shows marked oedema of most of the body, with ascites and pleural effusions due to hypoproteinaemia caused by the muscle mass being metabolized to produce energy. The dry form has little or no oedema, but there is hypotension and incipient cardiac failure.

The appearance in both the living and the dead is usually of a sunken, cachectic face, with skin stretched over the cheekbones and prominent jaw, zygoma and orbital margins. The eyes are sunken due to loss of orbital fat, though accompanying dehydration may also contribute to these appearances. The ribs, spine, iliac crests and all bony landmarks are prominent; the abdomen may be 'scaphoid' (i.e. concave between the costal margin and iliac crests) or it may be protuberant if ascites is a major factor. The diameter of the limbs is markedly reduced and the head may appear unduly large due to the narrowing of the neck. The skin may present various abnormalities. In children it is often pale and translucent, sometimes with a bluish tint due to the transparency of the tissues over veins. In the chronically starved, various skin diseases due to avitaminoses and infections may present as scaling, thickening or inflammatory lesions.

There may be pressure sores on the buttocks, sacrum and heels, due to loss of the padding effect of subcutaneous fat coupled with a reduction of skin viability and reduced mobility. There may be gum swelling, loosening of the teeth, sores on the lips and other signs of vitamin and protein deficiency, as well as infective lesions.

Internally, most organs except the brain may be reduced in weight compared to the normal range for age, sex and size. The stomach and intestines will commonly be distended with gas and appear thin walled and translucent. Occasionally, remnants of the ingested foreign material may be found in the stomach or bowel – in one case of a starved child, the remains of a paper nappy liner were found in all parts of the bowel. The gall bladder may be tense with bile due to lack of stimulus for emptying. There may be hard faecoliths in the rectum, but sometimes there is an enteritis with loose stools. There may be a smell of ketones on the breath and in the urine.

One of the medico-legal problems, especially when a child is alleged to have been denied proper feeding, is the possibility that some natural disease has caused the emaciated state. Full clinical investigations must then be made of either the living or the dead child, including an extensive radiological survey. An autopsy and histological survey are essential to confirm or refute the claim that conditions such as malignancy, Addison's disease, coeliac disease or a congenital metabolic defect are present.

Chapter twenty-two

General Aspects of Poisoning

In Britain, self-inflicted poisoning still accounts for a huge number of acute hospital consultations and admissions each day. Fortunately, only a minority of cases are fatal, but the cost to the health service is considerable.

The definition of poisoning can be difficult and it cannot be defined simply as an unwanted effect of ingestion of a chemical, because death is often the desired effect of ingesting the chemical in self-poisoning. It is perhaps better to discuss 'toxicity', which is simply the adverse effect of a chemical on cell, organ or organism from an objective viewpoint. Using this definition, virtually anything can be toxic if it is ingested in sufficient quantity and, in a chemical deliberately administered for treatment, it is the margin between any desired therapeutic effect and the adverse effects that is important.

Poisoning is very commonly accidental but, as noted above, a large number of cases are self-inflicted, often with the intention of committing suicide. Homicide by poison is now relatively rarely detected in advanced countries, despite the availability of well-equipped toxicology laboratories. The increasing cost of analysis and decreasing awareness of the problem of poisoning may have led to a false sense of complacency, which may in turn have led to the under-detection of poisoning from all causes. This has been clearly demonstrated recently in the UK by the murder of over 200 of his elderly patients by a general practitioner.

Accidental poisoning can vary from the individual case of a child eating medicinal tablets in mistake for sweets, to families dying from carbon monoxide due to a faulty gas appliance, to mass industrial disasters such as Bhopal in India, the leakage of dioxin gas in Italy and contaminated cooking oil in Spain. In warfare, the deliberate use of chemical weapons on a civilian population in Iraq and natural disasters such as the escape of carbon dioxide gas from a lake bed in Africa have claimed thousands of victims.

Agriculture is commonly associated with accidental poisoning because of the availability, often in a relatively uncontrolled environment, of toxic substances such as paraquat, organophosphorous insecticides etc. The history of toxicology is full of tragedies involving sacks of grain being left in rail-trucks contaminated with dieldrin, or of soft-drink bottles being re-filled with ethylene glycol anti-freeze or organophosphate weed killers. Other industrial processes are also associated with the use of potentially lethal chemicals: for example, the extraction of gold from ore and electroplating both use cyanide.

Suicidal poisoning is now the most common method of self-destruction for females and the second most common for males in England and Wales. The drugs and chemicals used depend upon their availability and upon some national and local practices. In Britain, there was a shift in the latter half of the twentieth century from barbiturates and aspirin to paracetamol,

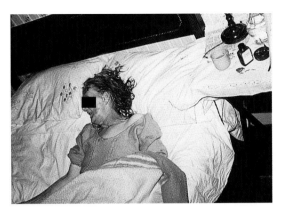

Figure 22.1 Drug overdosage must be considered when anyone is found dead unexpectedly and no fatal disease is discovered at autopsy.

then to the combination of paracetamol and dextropropoxyphene, and latterly to the tricyclic and other forms of antidepressants.

The suicidal use of corrosive agents has decreased dramatically compared with half a century ago, probably due to the availability of less painful alternatives. However, strong acids, alkalis or phenols or any other caustic or acidic substance may be drunk.

Homicidal poisoning is believed to be much less common than in the nineteenth century and it is also believed that this decrease is due to the decreased availability of toxic chemicals in society, because their manufacture, sale and use have been increasingly controlled by the state, rather than to a fundamental decline in the desire to commit homicide in this way. Where toxic substances are sold more freely, homicide by poison is by no means rare, and all manner of vegetable and inorganic toxins are used. The traditional weapons of the poisoner used to be the heavy metals such as arsenic and antimony or substances such as strychnine and cyanide. These are so easily detected by modern laboratory methods that they are now rarely used, though some surprising exceptions still occur.

THE TOXIC AND FATAL DOSE

There is a common misconception amongst the general public – but one that is also commonly found amongst police officers, lawyers, coroners and even some doctors – that for every drug or poison there is a fixed dose that will cause toxic symptoms and a larger dose that will kill. This simplistic view is utterly incorrect, as different people have a wide range of sensitivity (or resistance) to any given substance – and this sensitivity may vary from time to time in the same person.

The drug manufacturers have a broad test called the 'LD50' (lethal dose 50%), about which there is much confusion. The LD50 is the dose of a drug that will cause the death of half of the tested animals of a particular species in a series of experiments. Given that the population of animals will be expected to have a 'standard' distribution of responses to any drug, some animals will be alive and even apparently well on far higher doses than the LD50, whereas others will have died at much lower doses. If the LD50 cannot be used to predict the effect of a drug in an individual experimental animal, it certainly cannot be used to predict the effect of a drug on humans.

The concept of a minimum lethal dose is impossible to define for any one individual. However, when the large amounts of data collected by toxicology laboratories handling thousands of cases are analysed, a range can be determined within which most deaths and severe toxic effects will lie. Until quite recently, these data were accepted as being reliable. However, research has raised considerable concern about the use of data from autopsy material, as it has been found that errors due not only to the complex redistribution of chemicals in the fluid and tissue spaces of the body after death but also to simple sampling errors will lead to wide discrepancies in the levels of drug or chemical detected, even in the various parts of the same body. It has been shown that the post-mortem distribution of toxic substances is far from uniform, and so the drug concentration in blood taken from a peripheral vein is highly likely to be quite different from that in blood taken from the heart, great vessels or viscera. This is much less of a problem in the living, as the flowing circulation maintains a relatively uniform mixing – though it is well known, of course, that arterial and venous blood usually has different concentrations due to uptake by the tissues and organs.

It is difficult or impossible to 'back-calculate' from a blood concentration of a drug to try to estimate what dose was taken and at what time, and a medical witness would be well advised to avoid answering such a question. The problems here include:

- How long between taking the drug and death?
- What is the absorption rate of that drug? Is it constant?

- Is the drug completely absorbed from the alimentary canal?
- What is the rate of metabolism? Is it constant?
- What is the rate of excretion? Is it constant?
- Does the drug diffuse uniformly throughout all body tissues or does it vary between the aqueous, lipoid and other body compartments?
- Was the sample taken from an appropriate site?
- Has it been stored and analysed correctly?

TOLERANCE AND IDIOSYNCRASY

One of the problems of determining toxic or fatal doses of a drug or other chemical, and the equivalent blood levels, is that not only do different people have widely varying innate susceptibility, but tolerance can build up to a substance so that large doses no longer have the effect that they originally had. In analgesia, this tolerance, especially of the opiates, can cause therapeutic problems, as increasing doses need to be given to obtain the same beneficial effect. This can result in the administration of quantities of drugs that would normally be expected to cause death and the subsequent detection of greatly raised blood levels in individuals who are not only alive but conscious. This tolerance can develop rapidly, being established with some drugs within a couple of days or weeks, or it may take considerably longer. In evaluating toxicology results, the doctor has to take tolerance into account, as what may appear to be a toxic or fatal level in the blood or tissues may have had far less clinical effect than might be expected if tolerance has developed.

Tolerance is lost when exposure to the drug or chemical ceases, a fact that can have fatal results in the relapsing intravenous opiate drug abuser who, after a period of abstinence (either voluntary or enforced), returns to the same amount of drug and dies as a result. Generally speaking, the more rapidly tolerance develops, the more rapidly it will be lost. Many abused drugs – amphetamines, barbiturates, benzodiazepines and the morphine–heroin–methadone group – exhibit this phenomenon.

The opposite situation is that of idiosyncrasy, in which abnormally small amounts of substances – including penicillin, aspirin, cocaine and heroin – may cause dramatic or even fatal effects, some of which may be mediated by anaphylaxis and require previous exposure, whereas others induce a true idiosyncratic response on first exposure.

THE DOCTOR'S DUTY IN A CASE OF SUSPECTED POISONING

Whatever the cause or circumstances of poisoning, the medical attendant has a responsibility to manage the situation in the most effective way, by:

1 recognizing the fact or possibility of poisoning at the earliest possible stage;
2 instituting primary treatment and arranging admission to hospital when necessary;
3 identifying and retaining any drugs or possible poisons in the bedroom or household, workplace etc. and ensuring that these substances are taken to the treatment centre or hospital along with the patient so that they can be identified; and
4 where death has occurred, co-operating fully with the police, coroner, magistrate etc. in the investigation.

Commonly, an individual will present to a doctor in hospital with a history of accidental or deliberate poisoning, in which case the type(s) of drugs taken and when they were taken is crucial information. Diagnosis in an unconscious patient may depend as much on information from the scene as on physical examination of the body – empty tablet containers or 'blister packs' in the room or waste bins, notes describing intentions etc. are all important.

The recognition of concealed poisoning (whether accidental or homicidal) can be considerably more difficult, but the following symptoms and signs should at least cause the doctor to include poisoning in his first differential diagnosis:

- sudden vomiting and diarrhoea;
- unexplained coma, especially in children;
- coma in an adult known to have a depressive illness;
- rapid onset of a peripheral neuropathy, such as wrist-drop; and
- rapid onset of a neurological or gastrointestinal illness in someone known to be occupationally exposed to chemicals.

It is not all that uncommon for patients to allege that they are being poisoned (usually by a relative) or for a family member to allege that a recent death was due to poisoning. The majority of these claims are without any truth, and are due to misunderstandings, family feuds, malice, delusion or mental abnormality. In the living patient, the medical practitioner has first to decide whether the allegations may be true, based on his knowledge of the family situation and the personalities involved. If the signs and symptoms of the alleged victim are genuine and not inconsistent with some form of toxic effect, the doctor must take some steps to investigate and, in most instances, if the doctor has reason to believe the victim, he should advise him or her to inform the police so that a full investigation can be performed.

If there is real suspicion and cause for concern about the health of the victim, it would also make sense to remove the victim from the potential source of the poison, and this has been achieved in the past by admitting people to hospital or moving them to some other environment. It is then possible to monitor their symptoms and, if they clear up, this might suggest that some toxin was indeed being given. If an oral poison is suspected, friends and relatives should not be allowed to bring food or drink to the patient.

The possibility of deliberate self-administration of a poison for psychiatric reasons (Munchausen's syndrome) should always be borne in mind and, in children, the related problem of Munchausen's syndrome-by-proxy (in which one of the methods used by the carer to cause the child's illness is the administration of drugs or salt) has to be considered.

Samples for toxicological analysis, whether from clinical cases under investigation or under treatment or from autopsies, must be collected and stored with particular care. It is best practice that all samples must be meticulously labelled and identified at the time of removal or sampling, but this is an absolute necessity if there is any possibility of criminal action.

The doctor who takes a sample of blood from a venepuncture must place the blood into the appropriate tube and then immediately label it with the patient's name, address or hospital number, the date and preferably the time of sampling. The doctor's signature (or at least initials) should also be placed on the label. The tube will then usually be sealed into another receptacle such as a plastic bag, which may also be labelled with the details of the individual, the specimen and the person who took it. If the police are present (for instance at an autopsy), this sample will commonly be given a unique exhibit number. The doctor is the first person in what may be a long chain of custody of any specimen, and it is important for doctors to record in the medical notes what specimen(s) they took and at what time and to whom they gave the specimen and at what time.

This process is also called 'continuity of evidence' and every step in the chain from vein to laboratory must be capable of later proof in court if the opposing lawyers challenge the authenticity of the analysis. On no account should a specimen taken for these reasons be allowed to lie in a surgery, on a ward or elsewhere outside a sealed bag where it may be tampered with.

SAMPLES REQUIRED FOR TOXICOLOGICAL ANALYSIS

As to the nature of the preservation of samples, much depends upon the type of toxic substance suspected. The advice of the laboratory that is to carry out the analysis should be obtained, where there is any doubt, but the following is a generally accepted routine.

Blood

It is very important to obtain blood samples from the correct site. During life, any venous sample drawn from a limb vein is usually satisfactory, except in unusual circumstances when arterial blood is required. However, at autopsy, the site of sampling is of great importance because the interpretation of the results of analysis can be markedly distorted by an incorrect sample. The best place to obtain blood is from the femoral or iliac veins or, if no blood is available from those sites, from the axillary veins. The jugular venous system is not suitable as it may be contaminated by reflux from the upper thorax. Blood should never be taken from the general body cavity as it is highly likely to be grossly contaminated by intestinal contents, effusions, urine, faeces etc. Neither should blood be taken from the heart or great vessels in the chest as post-mortem diffusion of drugs and alcohol from the stomach or from aspirated vomit in the air passages can easily and rapidly contaminate the blood in these vessels. It has been shown, for example, that if fluid containing alcohol and paracetamol is instilled into the trachea after death to simulate aspiration of stomach contents, high blood concentrations of these substances can be detected in the thoracic vessels. Also, alcohol swallowed immediately before death, when it has had no time to be absorbed or to cause any physiological effects, can diffuse post mortem through the gastric wall into the blood in the heart and great vessel and so lead to a false-positive result on samples taken from these sites.

For most analyses, about 15 mL of blood from the iliac or femoral veins is placed in a plain tube, so that clotting can occur, together with 5–10 mL in a tube containing an anticoagulant, such as EDTA, potassium oxalate or heparin. In addition, an alcohol estimation is almost invariably required and 5 mL of blood for this should be placed in a sodium fluoride tube to inhibit production or destruction of alcohol by micro-organisms.

In autopsies upon victims of solvent abuse ('glue sniffers'), the chemical(s) responsible can often be recovered from the blood. Blood samples in cases of suspected solvent abuse should fill the bottle to the top so that there is no 'head space' into which the solvents can diffuse, only to be lost immediately on opening the bottle. It is far better to have a full small bottle in these cases than a half-empty large bottle.

Urine

Up to 20–30 mL of urine should be placed in a 'universal container'. No preservative is required unless there is to be a delay in reaching the laboratory. If this is so, then a small amount of sodium azide or fluoride can be added.

Vomit and stomach contents

If produced by a living patient or recovered from the scene of death, vomit may usefully be sent to the laboratory placed either in a clean glass jar or a plastic tub with a tight-fitting lid. At autopsy, the stomach contents may be saved into a similar container, by opening the greater curvature with scissors and allowing the contents to gravitate into the receptacle. Some laboratories also request the stomach wall itself, as powder and tablet debris may remain adherent to the mucosal folds in higher concentration.

Some well-organized toxicology laboratories provide kits consisting of a large and a small plastic tub, several universal containers, a fluoride tube, together with a syringe and needles and an instruction sheet, for use by doctors and pathologists.

Faeces

The contents of the rectum are not often required for analysis, except in suspected heavy-metal poisoning, such as arsenic, mercury or lead. A sample of 20–30 g should be taken into a plain screw-topped jar or a plastic container with a snap-on lid.

Liver and other organs

At autopsy, the most common organ to be saved for analysis is the liver, as higher concentrations of many drugs may be found, making them identifiable when the blood and urine concentrations have declined to very low or undetectable levels. The pathologist must examine the organ macroscopically for anatomical or pathological abnormalities and must sample it for microscopic examination before sending it for toxicological examination. Some laboratories request the whole organ, whereas others require only part of the liver. Whatever sample is required, it should be placed in a clean container. Some laboratories require the total weight of the organ, but this should routinely be noted as part of the internal examination and will be available if requested.

Bile is sometimes required for analysis and it is particularly useful for seeking evidence of chlorpromazine or morphine use.

Some laboratories analyse for solvents direct from an intact lung. In such a case, a lung should be taken straight from the body and placed in an impervious bag, which should be securely tied to avoid escape of vapour. Nylon bags, as used by arson investigators, are preferable to the usual polyvinyl chloride bags, as the latter are not completely impervious to organic solvents.

Hair and nail clippings

Heavy-metal poisonings by elements such as antimony, arsenic or thallium are often chronic events and some hair cut or pulled at the roots, together with nail clippings, should be submitted for analysis. These metals are laid down in keratin in a sequence depending on the time of administration, and it may even be possible, by neutron-activation analysis of a few hairs, to determine when in relation to the growth span of the hair the poison was administered, as the most recent doses will be nearer the root.

Recent advances in microchemistry have also allowed for the detection and analysis of opiate drugs in hair, and this can be used to confirm or refute prolonged drug use and even to identify approximately when (in terms of weeks or months) the drugs were used. Clearly, this is only of use if hair is present and is of sufficient length. The samples for this analysis should include the root to the tip of the hair, and the hairs should all be orientated in one direction.

Alcohol

Alcohol (ethyl alcohol, ethanol) is by far the most widely used drug in the world, even in those countries where religious beliefs theoretically prevent its consumption. Ethanol is a small, water-soluble molecule that becomes distributed evenly throughout the body water; it passes easily across the blood–brain barrier and has a profound depressant effect upon the cerebral function. It is a drug with huge morbidity and mortality, with direct toxic effects on the body tissues, but alcohol also has significant indirect effects and it is a very common catalyst in the majority of assaults and homicides. The use, or rather abuse, of alcohol pervades all aspects of legal medicine from the precipitation of many road traffic accidents and accidents at work through to professional misconduct of doctors, for whom alcohol abuse provides one of the most common reasons for disciplinary proceedings. Every medical practitioner needs to know something of the metabolism and effects of this ubiquitous substance.

SOURCES OF ALCOHOL

Ethanol is extremely easy to produce and almost all ethanol is produced by the action of yeast enzymes on vegetable substrates containing sugars. Direct (primary) fermentation cannot raise the concentration to more than 12–15 per cent, as the yeast is killed by the rising levels of alcohol. However, distillation of the primary fermentation can concentrate the alcohol to 40–60 per cent strength.

The usual forms of alcohol that are drunk have the following approximate strengths, excluding 'special' varieties, which are becoming more prevalent.

Beer, stout, cider	3–6%
Table wine	9–12%
Sherry, port (fortified with brandy)	17–21%
Spirits (whisky, brandy, gin, rum, vodka etc.)	35–45%

The concentration of alcohol must be written on the labels of most bottles containing it. It is usually written in the form of weight of alcohol per volume of liquid (w/v), rather than as volume of alcohol per volume of liquid, because alcohol has an appreciably lower specific gravity than water; for example 40% v/v whisky only has about 32 g per 100 mL. In order to simplify the understanding of the amount of alcohol consumed, the concept of a 'unit' of alcohol was introduced – a unit being about 8 g of alcohol – and in Britain this information is also on the labels of bottles. The following drinks all contain approximately 1 unit of alcohol.

Beer	half a pint (300 mL)
Wine	a 100-mL glass of table wine
Spirits	a small measure of spirits (25 mL)

It is generally stated that liver damage is unlikely if a man consumes fewer than 21 units per week, whereas a woman should consume fewer than 14 units per week to avoid liver damage.

ABSORPTION OF ALCOHOL

Most absorption of alcohol takes place in the stomach, duodenum and first part of the jejunum; the latter two are the most effective areas of absorption, partly because the gastric mucosa contains an alcohol dehydrogenase. Individuals with rapid stomach emptying or a gastro-jejunostomy may absorb alcohol unusually rapidly and this will produce a higher peak blood-alcohol concentration (BAC). A single bolus of alcohol taken into an empty stomach will be completely absorbed into the portal bloodstream within 30–90 minutes. As soon as alcohol enters the bloodstream, the liver and kidneys will begin to eliminate it, so the BAC achieved will be governed by the relative rates of absorption and elimination.

Absorption of alcohol is affected by:

- The presence of food in the stomach: food, especially fatty food, delays emptying through the pylorus, which will in turn delay contact with the mucosa of the more rapidly absorbing duodenal–jejunal segment of the intestines. Fatty food also physically obstructs the contact of alcohol molecules with the gastric mucosa.
- The concentration of alcohol: the optimum concentration for rapid absorption is about 20 per cent. The alcohol in weak drinks, such as beer, passes only slowly through the mucosa and into the bloodstream, whereas strong spirits irritate the gastric mucosa, resulting in the production of excess mucus, which will tend to coat the lining and produce a physical barrier to absorption. The pylorus may also undergo spasm, thus delaying gastric emptying and absorption.

ELIMINATION OF ALCOHOL

Well over 90 per cent of alcohol is metabolized by the liver, which accounts for the damaging effect that the long-term high intake of alcohol has upon that organ. Only 5–8 per cent of the alcohol is excreted unchanged by the kidneys, sweat and breath.

The rate of elimination from the bloodstream varies in different people: chronic alcoholics, particularly, who have induced liver cytochrome P450 enzymes (until their livers fail) can metabolize alcohol at an abnormally high rate. The 'normal' rate of elimination from the blood for non-alcoholics lies between about 11 and 25 mg/100 mL/h, with an average of 18 mg/100 mL/h; this can eliminate approximately 1 unit of alcohol (8 g) per hour.

THE MEASUREMENT OF ALCOHOL

The concentration of alcohol in both blood and urine is usually expressed in milligrams per hundred millilitres (mg/100 mL), sometimes written as mg/dL (decilitre). In some countries, as in the USA, the concentration is expressed as a percentage. The BAC is the most useful measure, because the rapid equilibration of alcohol across the blood–brain barrier means that the BAC reflects the concentration of alcohol currently affecting the brain.

The urine alcohol is more concentrated than the blood level, due to tubular resorption of water in the ratio of 1.3 : 1. However, it is less useful than blood-alcohol measurements, as the ureteric urine concentration varies with the rising or falling BAC and, as all the urine from the kidneys is pooled in the bladder, any sample of urine can only represent the mean value over the period of collection in the bladder.

Breath alcohol is in equilibrium with the alcohol in the blood, even though in a very small concentration of about 1 : 2300. At 37°C, a level of 1 mg/100 mL in blood will be equivalent to about 0.43 μg/100 mL in breath (and thus 1 μg/100 mL in breath is equivalent to about 2.28 mg/100 mL in blood). The exact ratio of blood alcohol/breath alcohol is temperature dependent and varies slightly with other factors such as the depth of respiration and the concentration of alcohol. Because the ratio is not constant, legal systems that use breath alcohol for detecting drinking drivers do not attempt to relate the breath level to the blood, but make the offence solely that of having exceeded a certain level in the breath itself.

THE EFFECTS OF ALCOHOL

Alcohol depresses the nervous system and any apparent initial excitant effect is due to suppression of inhibition by the cerebral cortex. The drug begins to act at the

Table 23.1 Guide to the Likely Effects of Alcohol on a Normal Adult

Blood-alcohol concentration (mg/dL)	Effects
30–50	Impairment of driving and similar skills
50–100	Reduced inhibitions, talkativeness, laughter, slight sensory disturbance
100–150	Incoordination, unsteadiness, slurred speech
150–200	Obvious drunkenness, nausea and ataxia
200–300	Vomiting, stupor, possibly coma
300–350	Danger of aspirating vomit, stupor or coma
350–450+	Progressive danger of death from respiratory paralysis

lowest concentrations upon the higher centres and it affects the lower centres of the central nervous system only when the BAC becomes higher. The effects of high levels of alcohol on the lower centres may jeopardize the function of the cardiorespiratory centres in the brainstem, with a consequent danger of death.

The earliest signs of alcohol intoxication can be found on objective testing with BAC as low as 30 mg/100 mL, when driving skills begin to deteriorate. Behaviour begins to change at a very variable level, but this is also influenced by emotional and environmental factors. A person is likely to appear more uninhibited in a student party than in a very formal function given the same level of alcohol.

The guide in Table 23.1 is a reasonable summation, given the great variations, in relation to the effects of alcohol in blood.

To illustrate the uncertainty of this type of table, in Australia, numerous drunken drivers have been found to have BACs of over 500 mg/100 mL, when they should technically be dead, and people have survived alcohol concentrations of over 1500 mg/100 mL (albeit with medical support in intensive care) – these individuals are almost always chronic alcoholics.

DANGERS OF DRUNKENNESS

Apart from the danger of respiratory paralysis at high concentrations of alcohol, there are many other hazards (some of which can be fatal), which can beset the drunken person. Accidents of all types are more common: individuals under the influence of drink fall down and frequently suffer injuries, especially to their heads; falls down stairs or steps and into the roadway are common and people who are under the influence of alcohol are more likely to be pedestrian victims of road traffic accidents.

Drinking and personal violence are a common combination and altercations, fights and assaults are a frequent sequel to intoxication, with all the possible injurious and fatal consequences.

Burns are another possibility and typically occur when a drunken person falls asleep in bed while smoking a cigarette, which may be dropped into the bedding, death ensuing from burns or carbon monoxide inhalation. Drowning is another common sequel, particularly in seamen and others who work or live around ships or docks, as they fall from quays, gangways and decks when unsteady due to drink.

Vomiting is not uncommon in those intoxicated by alcohol, due to the irritant effect of alcohol upon the gastric mucosa. Vomiting combined with decreased laryngeal reflexes allows the irritant gastric contents to enter the airways, where they may cause death by stimulation of the vagus nerve, with resultant cardiac depression, or by simple mechanical obstruction.

The police are most commonly left to deal with those members of the community who cause a disturbance or otherwise offend the public after consuming too much alcohol. The police have few places to put these people, other than in a cell in a police station. Although most police forces have a strict regime for placing inebriated individuals in a semi-prone position and inspecting them at frequent intervals, deaths of these people while in custody are not uncommon and represent a disaster – for the family, for the police and for society. It is interesting to note that we do not place an individual with any other form of drug abuse into custody simply because they are under the influence of that drug, and many deaths would be prevented each year if these cases were treated in the same way as other types of acute poisoning.

Alcohol-induced disease is extremely common and an appreciable proportion of national medical care is consumed by drink-related conditions. Liver disease is due to progressive damage to the hepatic cells caused by high concentrations of alcohol and its breakdown products. Fatty change is common following the ingestion of alcohol, although at low levels it may be apparent only microscopically. Continued ingestion of alcohol will be followed by fibrosis, which, if it becomes sufficiently extensive, is then termed cirrhosis. Once cirrhosis is established, a series of clinical events will follow, including splenomegaly, portal hypertension with the development of varices and possibly gastrointestinal bleeding.

Liver function tests will assist in monitoring the condition of the liver and a specific enzyme marker is gamma-glutamyl transpeptidase (GGT), which is elevated well above 36 units in alcoholic liver damage. Alcohol also affects the brain in long-term alcoholics, even when full-blown Wernicke's encephalopathy is not present. The myocardium also suffers and although there are no definite histological criteria for alcoholic cardiomyopathy, there is no doubt of its existence as a clinical entity. Alcohol is also the cause of considerable fetal abnormality and the features of the fetal alcohol syndrome are well defined.

DRINKING AND DRIVING

This is a major problem all over the world, even in Islamic countries where alcohol is officially banned. Even small quantities of alcohol impair driving efficiency and objective testing, demonstrating deterioration of skills at a BAC of only 30 mg/100 mL. Some countries, such as in Eastern Europe, have a zero limit for driving, but elsewhere the threshold of blood or breath concentration varies considerably.

For example, the countries of the British Isles have a BAC limit of 80 mg/100 mL in blood, 35 mg/100 mL in breath or 107 mg/100 mL in urine. This is thought to be too high by the British Medical Association, which wishes the government to bring the limit down to 50 mg/100 mL in blood. However, it must be admitted that over half the drivers charged with excess alcohol have more than twice the legal limit in their breath or blood, so reducing the lower limit would be irrelevant in their case.

The role of the doctor in the investigation of drinking and driving varies according to the method of enforcement used in a particular country. Where there is no statutory limit by blood or breath, a doctor may have to carry out clinical testing of the driver to decide if his ability to control the vehicle is impaired. This can be a very subjective decision in marginal cases, although the evidence of blood and breath testing

shows that many drinking drivers are so far 'over the limit' that a decision as to their condition is not difficult. Where a statutory limit is part of the law, some countries require blood samples to be taken by a doctor by venepuncture, whereas others, including Britain, accept evidential breath testing performed by trained police officers. If urine is used in place of blood or breath, it can also be collected by police officers.

In addition to testing for driving ability, a doctor may be required to examine a suspected drunken driver to exclude or confirm natural disease or injury that may mimic alcoholic intoxication. Diabetic precoma, insulin overdose with hypoglycaemia, carbon monoxide poisoning from a leaking exhaust system, a head injury and many other disease processes have to be considered in this examination. Another problem is the impairment of driving ability from drugs other than alcohol – either medicinal substances or drugs of dependence – and this has been the subject of recent research in the UK.

Scheme of examination for impairment of ability to drive

This is an examination not to discover if the driver is in a drunken state but to decide whether his ability to control a vehicle safely is impaired for whatever reason. Unless the examination also includes the taking of samples for blood, breath or urine for analysis, its value in confirming alcoholic intoxication is limited, except when the subject is obviously inebriated. Informed consent to the examination is essential and the driver must be aware that the facts may be used in criminal proceedings. If the person refuses permission, no attempt should be made forcibly to examine him, as this would be an assault. However, the person can be observed and a report offered on that basis. If the subject is too drunk to understand or give consent, only the results of observation can be provided to the police. In these circumstances, it may also be necessary, for the person's own safety, to perform some examination to exclude serious injury and to protect him from the potential dangers of severe drunkenness. Even when consent has been obtained, the driver may wish a doctor of his own choice to be present on his behalf; this is quite acceptable but it must not so delay the examination that the intoxication passes off or is significantly reduced. The British Medical Association has recommended that no more than half an hour should elapse.

The examination begins with history taking, especially about past medical history and the taking of any medicines or drugs, especially insulin, oral hypoglycaemic agents, sedatives, anti-epileptic drugs, antihistamines (which might produce drowsiness) and other hypnotics or tranquillizers. This is not only relevant to the present examination, but also gives the doctor an opportunity to assess coherence of speech, confusion, memory and general mental ability. The demeanour, whether excited, depressed, drowsy or aggressive etc., is recorded. The amount, type and timing of the person's recent drinking should be determined as well as some idea of his long-term drinking habits. The quantities admitted by the person should be noted – but not necessarily believed!

General tests of memory and mental alertness may be incorporated into the history taking, unless the driver is obviously drunk, when simple direct questions about the date and time may have to be asked.

The subject should then be asked to write something either from dictation or copied from a book or paper, but in making this assessment the doctor should allow for the apparent social and educative standard of the person: many may be unable to write well or at all, even when sober, in which case drawing simple patterns, such as triangles and diamonds, may be preferable. Simple tests of dexterity such as picking up small objects from the floor are preferable to walking a chalk-line on the floor, which even sober people often cannot perform well.

When undressing for examination, the ability to undo buttons, any fumbling with zips etc. should be noted. The physical examination should follow a normal medical routine, seeking physical evidence of natural disease or injury. The scalp should be inspected and palpated for evidence of any head injury. The eyes should be carefully examined, seeking evidence of visual acuity, such as reading the time on a clock across a room. The full range of eye movements, nystagmus, strabismus and pupil reactions must be tested. Lateral nystagmus must be distinguished from nystagmoid jerks due to the examiner's finger moving beyond the field of vision.

The condition of the skin should be noted – dry, cold, sweaty or flushed. The pulse rate and volume and the blood pressure are to be taken. In intoxication, the skin may be warm and flushed, as are the conjunctivae. The pulse is full and bounding.

The smell of the breath may confirm that alcohol has been taken and, on occasion, the type of drink, but is no guide whatsoever to the amount. If blood is to be taken, the antecubital fossa of the elbow is the chosen site. It is vital when cleaning the skin not to use any antiseptic that contains alcohol. Some proprietary pre-packed swabs have ethanol as a solvent and even the slightest hint of vapour from these swabs on the skin may totally distort the analytical result.

About 5 mL of blood are taken into a tube containing sodium fluoride, with or without potassium oxalate as an anticoagulant. The tube is thoroughly mixed by inversion and carefully labelled with the driver's details and countersigned by the doctor. If it cannot immediately be sent for analysis, it should be kept at ordinary refrigerator temperature (5 °C, not deep-frozen) until despatch. In many jurisdictions, two samples are taken for the laboratory and a third is offered to the driver in case he wishes to have his own sample analysed by an independent laboratory.

If urine is to be taken, the driver should empty his bladder completely and then, after 30 or 60 minutes, they should be asked to provide a specimen direct into a clean and sterile container.

Breath samples are usually taken by trained police officers and are rarely the concern of the doctor.

The report on the examination should be written at the time and, at the end of the examination, the police should be informed of the doctor's opinion, as they will have to make decisions about whether to charge the driver and also whether he is fit to be detained in the police station, whether he can be allowed to return to his vehicle or whether he must be admitted to hospital.

If a driver is admitted to hospital after an accident, the decision to allow a doctor employed by the police to examine him rests with the hospital clinician. The clinician must decide if the clinical state of the driver is satisfactory enough for this to be done, but the doctor must not use clinical freedom to shelter someone who might be a continuing danger to the public. If it is desired to take blood for alcohol analysis from a driver in hospital, he must give permission: it is not ethical (unless the law of that country allows it) to use a blood sample taken for clinical diagnostic purposes for alcohol analysis without the consent of the patient. If he is unconscious, the sample must be kept until he is able to decide on consent.

Drugs of Dependence and Abuse

Drug abuse is a worldwide problem with numerous manifestations: from the 'drug cartel' assassinations in South America to the prostitutes in the cities of Europe, to the pathetic death of a solitary drug user in a public toilet of any city, town or village. The dead solitary drug abuser represents the commonest face of drug abuse, but it is a problem that affects all strata of society and is not confined to the dirty and the destitute. A doctor may self-prescribe analgesics and middle-class, middle-aged women are not uncommonly addicted to benzodiazepines. It is essential for a forensic practitioner to know about the major drugs of dependence and abuse and to be able to recognize the signs and symptoms of drug abuse on physical examination of either the living or dead.

Drugs may be taken by injection (intravenous, subcutaneous or, rarely, intramuscular), by sniffing (snorting) into the nose, by inhalation or orally. The different routes of ingestion may produce different physical lesions. It is very rare for drugs to be abused by the vaginal or rectal route, but large amounts of drugs may be transported, wrapped, in these orifices. In general, most drug users will appear perfectly normal; the popular image of an emaciated wreck covered in septic sores is true only in a very small minority.

In those who do exhibit some physical abnormality, it is usually not due to the drugs themselves, but rather to the associated complications of the prolonged use of the drugs: general ill-health, loss of weight due to anorexia or simple lack of money for food. The lack of a suitable diet may lead to avitaminosis and intercurrent infections in addition to the more specific infections directly related to drug usage.

TOLERANCE AND SYNERGY

Most of the commonly abused drugs, such as heroin, cocaine, methadone, amphetamines and barbiturates, invoke 'tolerance', which is not the same, or even linked to, dependence. Tolerance means that a dose of a drug does not produce the 'normal' or 'standard' physical or psychological effects. Natural tolerance is genetically determined (fewer receptor sites, increased enzyme activity etc.) and it is not due to previous use of the drug. Acquired tolerance depends upon previous exposure to the drug and may be due to a number of factors, including reduced sensitivity of receptor sites or induction of metabolic enzymes. Rapidly developing tolerance is known as tachyphylaxis. Cross-tolerance for other chemically similar drugs is common and, surprisingly, tolerance can also be demonstrated between chemically dissimilar compounds (e.g. alcohol and barbiturates). Increasing dosages mean that any dose-related toxic side-effects also increase and, because more drug needs to be taken, the social consequences are also magnified and so more money is needed to buy the drugs.

The opposite of cross-tolerance is synergy, when one drug increases the effects of another, either by summation (alcohol and ether) or by potentiation (amphetamine and monoamine oxidase inhibitors).

DEPENDENCE AND WITHDRAWAL SYMPTOMS

Dependence, on the other hand, means the inability of the user to give up the habit, and dependence goes hand in hand with tolerance to worsen the vicious circle that is soon established. Dependence to some drugs can develop very quickly and some authorities would go so far as to claim that even a single exposure to some potent drugs is sufficient to 'hook' some recipients.

When the drugs are withdrawn, due either to attempts at treatment or to the inability to sustain the habit, severe symptoms can sometimes develop. These symptoms are sometimes called 'cold turkey', but this terminology is most commonly used in relation to the most common variety – opiate withdrawal. Placebos can reduce the symptoms of withdrawal for a while and the withdrawal 'syndrome' is, for the most part, psychological, but it also has some genuinely physiological aspects. The symptoms of acute withdrawal include fear and anxiety, muscle twitching, yawning, sweating, lacrimation, tremors, 'gooseflesh' of the skin and cramps, which may be followed by diarrhoea and incontinence. Restlessness and insomnia accompany tachycardia and hypertension.

THE DANGERS OF DRUG DEPENDENCE

Complications of injections

The repeated injection of drugs damages the peripheral veins wherever they are used, most commonly in the arms, hands and legs but sometimes in the groin or neck, and repeated use of the same vein or group of veins leads to phlebitis and thrombosis, especially if the injected substance is either irritant or non-sterile. On examination, it is possible to see that the veins eventually become dark in colour under the skin and

may feel hard and cord-like due to thrombosis and fibrosis; the overlying skin may even ulcerate. Skin abscesses, which may extend deep into the subcutaneous tissues and depressed areas of fat atrophy, may complicate sites of intravenous drug abuse and there is often fat necrosis and, with deep injection sites, chronic myositis. When healed, the superficial multiple puncture sites along a vessel may result in linear, white or silvery scars lying along the axis of the limb. There are numerous other complications, including septicaemia and subacute bacterial endocarditis, which may occur where pyogenic organisms are injected or enter the bloodstream from abcesses and other sites of infection.

Other complications of drug dependence are pulmonary tuberculosis and pneumonias, which develop from a combination of increased exposure to the infective organisms due to poor living conditions and reduced resistance and poor nutrition.

SHARED SYRINGES

The use of shared syringes and needles between groups of addicts can transmit hepatitis B and C, HIV virus and even malaria. In many countries, needle and syringe swap schemes have been introduced to reduce this risk.

SOLID DRUGS

Tablets are crushed or capsules are opened and the solid contents are then dissolved in water, commonly with a little citric acid to acidify the water and using some heat from a lighter or candle. The water may be clean but is very seldom sterile and, more commonly, it is from a highly contaminated source such as a toilet. The solution obtained is drawn up into a syringe and then injected. Any undissolved fragments of drug or tablet filler will become impacted in the capillary beds and commonly lead to micro-emboli in the lungs and liver. Birefringent material (commonly the starch filler from the tablets) and granulomas can often be seen on microscopic examination of the lungs and there may also be a wide spectrum of pulmonary changes, from acute abscesses to chronic fibrosis, associated with these debris emboli.

OVERDOSAGE AND HYPERSENSITIVITY

Deaths may occur very rapidly, especially with the intravenous use of heroin; indeed, death may be so rapid that the needle and syringe may still be in the vein when the body is found. A few of the deaths of 'first-time users' may be due to some personal hypersensitivity to the drug. However, the relative lack of hypersensitivity when using heroin or other opiates clinically suggests that if hypersensitivity does occur, it is more likely that it is to some contaminant in the material that was injected rather than to the drug itself. Habituated users are not immune to sudden death. This may be due to hypersensitivity on the basis of previous exposure, but it may also be due to taking an excessive amount of drug, either deliberately or accidentally, because a different supply has less diluent cut into it and so the same amount of powder contains a greater amount of active drug.

The post-mortem features are commonly those of acute left ventricular failure with gross pulmonary oedema, which may rarely be apparent on external examination as a plume of froth exuding from the mouth and nose.

The need to obtain money to sustain the drug habit may lead to squalor, theft and prostitution. Drug abusers are much more likely to be involved in accidents of all kinds, including traffic accidents, falls and fires, because of their impaired awareness and behaviour and also because of the environment in which many live. Personal violence and murder are also much more common. Death can also occur from poisonous contaminants (strychnine etc.) that have been used, accidentally or deliberately, to dilute the drugs.

HEROIN, MORPHINE AND OTHER OPIATES

Opiates, both naturally occurring and synthetic, are very common drugs of abuse, heroin being preferred by addicts due to its more intense action. Pure morphine is rarely used in urban drug dependence; it is poorly absorbed from the gut and so is usually injected or smoked as opium, especially in Asia. Other opioid drugs include codeine (di-methyl morphine), dihydrocodeine (DF 118), papaverine (Omnopon), pethidine, dipipanone, methadone, dextromoramide, pentazocine, cyclizine, diphenoxylate, propoxyphene and dextropropoxyphene. Most of these are legitimate

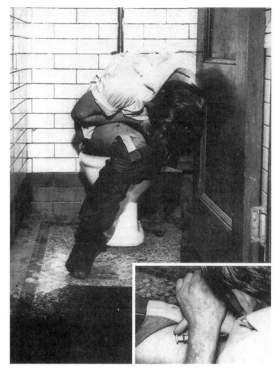

Figure 24.1 Death of a heroin abuser in a public toilet. The needle is still in the vein.

pharmacological substances but find their way onto the illicit market.

Solid heroin (di-acetyl morphine) can be either dissolved in a liquid (see above) that is then injected or it can be heated (usually on a piece of silver foil) and the smoke or vapour inhaled ('chasing the dragon'). Opiates are central nervous system depressants and heroin causes excitation by lifting cortical inhibitions in a similar manner to alcohol. Opiates soon induce tolerance, so that increasing doses must be used for the same effect.

The signs of opiate toxicity commonly include pinpoint pupils, sweating, warm skin, low blood pressure and slow breathing, which may progress to respiratory arrest if the dosage is high enough. Heroin can also cause sudden death, but the exact mechanism involved in any individual case will probably remain obscure unless admission to hospital and clinical monitoring have occurred. Even people who have been abusing the drug for some time may be found dead, and sometimes it is clear that they have died extremely rapidly. Severe pulmonary oedema is the common autopsy finding and this has probably developed from a sudden ventricular dysrhythmia.

Pethidine is more excitant than hypnotic and appears to have an atropine-like effect, with dilated pupils, tachycardia and dry mouth. Monoamine oxidase inhibitors and phenothiazines can produce severe reactions and even death when taken in conjunction with pethidine.

Methadone was introduced as a less dangerous alternative to heroin and was used in substitution treatment for heroin addiction in an effort to reduce dependence. However, it has become a drug of addiction in its own right and in some places it is claimed that more deaths occur from methadone than from the drugs it was intended to replace.

Dipipanone is an analgesic drug, often combined with cyclizine under the trade name Diconal, which has also become a widely used drug of abuse.

BARBITURATES AND OTHER HYPNOTICS

In terms of sheer quantity, barbiturates used to be by far the most common addictive drugs, but stringent controls on dispensing and prescribing together with changing fashions have seen a marked reduction in their use. A wide range of compounds is available, from the short-acting anaesthetic drugs such as thiopentone sodium through to the medium-acting amylobarbitone. The long-acting barbiturates such as phenobarbitone are now only used in the treatment of epilepsy in humans, but they are still widely available as veterinary products. Tolerance is rapidly induced and withdrawal symptoms can be severe. Barbiturates ('downers') may be combined with stimulant amphetamines ('uppers') in the same tablet, once known as a 'purple heart'. Alcohol and barbiturates have a powerful additive action and have been responsible for many deaths.

AMPHETAMINES

Amphetamine (benzedrine) and dextroamphetamine (dexedrine) were originally prescribed to delay fatigue and for appetite suppression; they have a strong stimulant effect, which in chronic use may lead to hyperexcitement, hallucinations and psychoses. Commonly, there is hyperpyrexia and hypertension, which can occasionally precipitate a cerebral or subarachnoid haemorrhage, and there is also a risk of cardiac arrhythmias.

MDMA (methylene-dioxy-methamphetamine) – also known also as 'Ecstasy', 'XTC' or 'ADAM' – which appeared a number of years ago as a 'designer drug', has been responsible for a number of deaths. Its use in Western countries is now widespread, especially amongst teenagers as an aid to 'rave' activities such as all-night dancing. It is said that, in 1996, probably a third of young people in Britain had used 'Ecstasy', with appreciable morbidity and some mortality. MDMA use may result in neurological, renal, hepatic and pulmonary complications and, in addition, rhabdomyolysis and disseminated intravascular coagulation may be present. Some users have been known to drink large quantities of water, which may result in water intoxication and death from cerebral oedema.

COCAINE

This substance, known for centuries through the effects of consumption of the coca leaf in South America, is a competitor for heroin (with which it may be combined) as the largest-volume drug of abuse. Cocaine is either inhaled into the nostrils or injected, though some is smoked. Ulceration of the nasal septum is always recorded as a complication of long-term nasal abuse of cocaine but this is, in fact, a rare phenomenon.

When cocaine usage is suspected during a medical examination or an autopsy, cotton-wool swabs from each nostril should be sent for laboratory analysis. Tolerance is rapidly developed and the user requires larger and larger doses for the same excitant effect. Abuse of cocaine is said to be followed by profound depression and may lead to severe mental dysfunction. Unlike the opioids, there are few physical withdrawal symptoms.

Cocaine produces hypertension, which (like amphetamines) may lead to cerebral bleeding. Dilated pupils, hyperpyrexia, marked sweating and confusion may lead to coma and death from either respiratory depression or cardiac arrhythmia. In the last few years, an allegedly more potent form of cocaine called 'crack' has appeared; it is made by heating cocaine together with an alkali such as bicarbonate. The name arises from the noise made when it is being prepared as well as the fissured appearance of the heated cocaine. Increased rapidity of action and heightened effect are claimed for 'crack', and this is said to be associated with an increase in the speed of development of dependence.

Cocaine is also known to have chronic effects upon a number of organs, particularly the heart, which may show foci of scarring that may themselves be the source of fatal dysrhythmias, even in the absence of circulating cocaine. Ingestion of cocaine is also associated with the development of an unusual but potentially fatal state of over-excitement called excited delirium. The bizarre behaviour exhibited in this state may result in attempts at restraint by the police and many sudden deaths have been recorded in these circumstances.

CANNABIS

Under a wide variety of names, such as hashish, bhang, hemp, marihuana, ganja etc., cannabis is used throughout much of the world, either smoked or by mouth. It never causes death and its dangers are denied by many, though long-term users may develop psychotic states and there is some evidence of genetic defects in the offspring of users.

LYSERGIC ACID DIETHYLAMIDE (LSD)

This hallucinogenic substance, which is not addictive, was commonly used in the 1960s. It was associated with a number of deaths because of accidents during the so-called 'trip', as distortion of perception persuaded the users that they could fly from high windows or stop passing buses with their bare hands. The hallucinations and visual disturbances associated with this drug can be terrifying ('bad trip') and some users have developed frankly psychotic states resembling schizophrenia. The tiny (microgram) doses needed meant that LSD could be circulated with relative impunity, carried in a single drop soaked into a lump of sugar or a scrap of blotting paper.

Other hallucinogenic drugs include mescaline, originally extracted from a Mexican cactus, and psilocybin, a drug obtained from the 'magic mushrooms' that are collected and dried on a large scale in Europe.

More dangerous is phencyclidine, nick-named 'angel dust' or PCP (an acronym of its chemical name, phenyl-cyclohexyl-piperidine). This can be injected, inhaled or smoked, often in conjunction with other drugs. It produces hyperexcitability, often aggressive, and has led to many deaths, some of them suicidal or homicidal.

SOLVENT ABUSE

During the 1980s and 1990s, a new form of addictive or dependent behaviour emerged, which was originally called 'glue sniffing' because the most widely used substance that contained the active compound – toluene – was an adhesive. The practice is still common, although much less publicized in the UK. It is said to be most frequent in older children and teenagers, boys outnumber girls and 90 per cent of the deaths are in males under the age of 30. It has been claimed that between 3.5 and 10 per cent of British teenagers have experimented with the habit.

Toluene is not the only substance abused and nowadays a wide variety of volatile substances is used, most of which are organic solvents, giving the name to the syndrome.

The usual way in which these substances are used is by placing some of the solvent-containing material in a plastic bag and holding the open end over the nose and mouth. Alternatively, the pure solvent is soaked onto a handkerchief or rag and the vapour is inhaled. Both methods give the desired effect of intoxication and hallucination.

Volatiles such as paint stripper, typewriting erasing fluid, brush cleaner, household aerosols, fabric cleaner, gasoline as well as glue solvents are misused in this way, as are many common materials that contain substances such as ethylene chloride, carbon tetrachloride, benzene, halon, trichloethane, toluene, xylene and trichlorethylene.

Another variation is the use of gases, such as butane, propane and bromo-fluoro-carbons. These can be obtained from cylinders for cigarette-lighter refills and cooking stoves and from fire extinguishers. The gas, under high pressure, may be sprayed directly into the mouth for inhalation, sometimes causing sudden death, perhaps from vagal stimulation by the freezing gas.

Death in any form of solvent abuse may be sudden and unexpected and from a variety of causes. The direct use of gas has been mentioned, but many of the solvents seem to sensitize the myocardium to catecholamines (adrenaline and noradrenaline) so that, even after the sniffing has ceased, any sudden fright that releases catecholamines can precipitate ventricular fibrillation and cardiac arrest. Vomit entering the air passages, sheer hypoxia (especially if the plastic bag is placed over the head) or a direct toxic effect of the substance on the tissues, especially the brain and myocardium, are alternative mechanisms.

Little is found on examination of these victims, although if glue has been used frequently, there may be sores and excoriations on the lips, and microscopic damage to the cells of the liver, cerebral and cerebellum may occur. If solvent abuse is suspected, blood samples taken for toxicology must fill the container so that the solvent is not lost from the 'head space' when the lid is removed. Organ samples must be placed in nylon bags to prevent loss of the solvent during transportation to the laboratory.

Chapter twenty-five

Medicinal Poisons

Analgesics	Barbiturates	Phenacetin	Insulin
Antidepressant and sedative drugs	Chloral	Lithium	

Almost any pharmaceutical substance is potentially poisonous if taken in sufficient dosage or for a long period. However, toxic and fatal consequences are most commonly accidental or suicidal, although homicide should always be borne in mind, even though it is rare.

It is impossible in a book of this size to mention more than a few drugs of particular forensic interest; however, there is great variation in the drugs prescribed, used and, most importantly, available to the public in different countries. In many countries, there are strict controls on the supply of drugs but many potentially lethal compounds are still available to the public without prescription in the shops. In other countries, most drugs can be easily bought from chemists without the need for a prescription. In less-developed countries, the availability and cost of drugs are the main limiting factors and so few drugs are available, either with or without a prescription. Where drugs are easily available, they are by far the most common method of suicide and suicidal gestures. The drugs used and the other 'fashions' in self-poisoning vary with place and time; for example aspirin overdose used to be common in Britain and rare in continental Europe, and barbiturates were once the most frequent cause of fatal overdose in Britain, yet both have declined markedly and paracetamol (acetaminophen) is now one of the most common agents used in suicide. In countries where pharmaceutical drugs are rare, it follows that overdoses using these drugs will

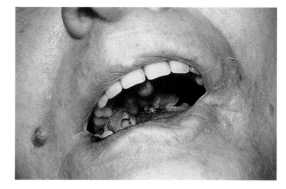

Figure 25.1 An overdose of drugs may, rarely, still be in the mouth.

also be rare and other methods of suicide will be more common.

The autopsy appearances in most medicinal poisonings are usually unhelpful unless corrosive or irritative substances are ingested (which is now rare) or identifiable tablet residues are present in the mouth or stomach. The diagnosis depends on the history, the circumstances and the results of the analysis of body fluids and tissues.

The following groups of drugs and individual compounds are representative of the dangerous usage of pharmaceuticals, but the subject has expanded so greatly that it properly belongs in the field of clinical toxicology rather than legal medicine, and a textbook should be consulted if more detailed information is required.

ANALGESICS

These include codeine, paracetamol (acetaminophen), aspirin, dichlorophenazone, dextropropoxyphene, acetanilide, phenazone, phenylbutazone, amidopyrine, ibuprofen etc. Many combined preparations such as distalgesic or coproxamol, both of which contain both paracetamol and dextropropoxyphene, are also available and many are sold without prescription.

Aspirin is acetyl-salicylic acid, often modified into less irritant forms such as soluble aspirin or calcium aspirin. It was once a favoured drug for suicide and particularly for suicidal 'gestures'. Its toxicity varies greatly in different people, some having virtually no symptoms after taking a hundred 300-mg tablets, whereas others with some rare idiosyncratic sensitivity to the substance will die after ingesting only a few tablets. These latter victims usually suffer a hypersensitivity reaction with urticaria, angio-neurotic oedema, hypotension, vasomotor disturbances and laryngeal and glottal oedema. Deaths in adults can occur after taking between 25 and 50 tablets if no treatment is given. In children, a quarter of that dose can be very dangerous and an association of aspirin with Reye's syndrome has led to a ban on the administration of this drug to children under 12 years, except in very specific circumstances.

In many people, large doses of aspirin lead to vomiting, which beneficially removes much of the drug from the stomach, but even if they retain a large amount of the drug, they suffer no effects at all or they suffer only from a range of symptoms related to the metabolic effects of the acidic aspirin, including ringing in the ears, dizziness, faintness, air hunger, pallor and sweating. Occasionally, hyperventilation and coma might ensue. A particular danger, even where symptoms are mild or even absent, is the onset of cardiac arrhythmias and sudden death, and this risk persists for a day or so after the overdose. Aspirin is a potent anticoagulant and some bleeding disorders can follow overdose; gastric haemorrhage is not uncommon, especially as the solid compound can erode the gastric mucosa when in close contact. At autopsy on fatal cases, multiple haemorrhagic foci may be seen in the gut and on serosal surfaces in the thorax.

Patients who are on long-term salicylate therapy for rheumatic disorders may have blood levels in excess of those seen in some fatal overdoses, which makes interpretation of toxicological results difficult.

For example, patients on 3 g aspirin per day may have blood concentrations as high as 300 mg/L – fatal levels vary between about 60 and 750 mg/L, with a mean level at around 500 mg/L.

As already mentioned, paracetamol is now the most common cause of self-administered overdosage in Britain. The drug is often taken in one of the combination preparations also containing dextropropoxyphene, which will cause death before the toxic effects of the paracetamol are apparent. Paracetamol is used therapeutically in doses of up to 1 g per day; overdoses of 20 g or more are potentially fatal. Paracetamol is a potent hepatic toxin, a small part being converted by the mixed function oxidase system (P450) into N-acetyl-p-benzoquinoneimine (NAPQI); normally glutathione and other sulphydryl compounds detoxify this substance. In overdose, the detoxification mechanism is overloaded and the NAPQI accumulates sufficiently to cause a severe centrilobular liver necrosis. This is a relatively slow but inexorable process if sufficient drug has been taken and most paracetamol deaths are delayed for several days until liver failure occurs.

Typical blood levels in overdoses of about 10–15 g are in the region of 100–400 mg/L and the toxicological analysis of blood levels provides a good guide to the value of treatment and the ultimate prognosis. A graph of paracetamol concentration against time since ingestion can be used to determine if treatment with intravenous acetylcysteine or oral methionine is required. As a rough guide, 4 hours after ingestion a paracetamol level of more than 200 mg/L (1.3 mmol/L) requires treatment; this falls to 100 mg/L at 8 hours and 50 mg/L at 12 hours. It has now been noted that certain individuals are considered to be at higher risk of developing hepatic necrosis with paracetamol. This group includes those with anorexia and alcoholism and those who are HIV positive as well as those taking enzyme-inducing drugs, including phenytoin, phenobarbital, carbamazepine and rifampicin.

Rarely, a massive overdose results in a quite rapid death from direct effects on the brainstem. At autopsy, liver damage and sometimes an associated renal tubular necrosis may be the only findings.

Ibuprofen is one of a large group (naproxen, fenbrufen etc.) of the newer non-steroidal anti-inflammatory drugs (NSAIDs) that are derived from propionic acid; other members of the NSAID group (diclofenac, phenylbutazone, mefenamic acid etc.) are derived from other sources. The effects of overdoses are as variable as the members of the NSAID group. In general, there may be some local gastrointestinal symptoms and some members of the group are associated with some aspirin-like symptoms, but these drugs are better therapeutically and safer when taken in excess than aspirin.

ANTIDEPRESSANT AND SEDATIVE DRUGS

Though relatively innocuous, the antidepressants (prescribed in huge quantities in many parts of the world) can cause toxic symptoms and even death in overdose. The tricyclic group, amitriptyline, dothiepin, trimipramine (which also have a sedative action) and imipramine, nortriptyline, desipramine etc., and the tetracyclic antidepressants, including maprotiline and mianserin, commonly have anticholinergic actions and, though relatively safe in therapeutic dosage, at the high levels in overdose they can cause death from brainstem depression with respiratory failure, convulsions and sudden cardiac arrhythmias.

Selective serotonin re-uptake inhibitor (SSRI) drugs form the latest group of antidepressant drugs and include fluoxetine, paroxetine and sertraline. Hypersensitivity reactions and side-effects can occur and, although the drugs are relatively safe, deaths have been reported with ingestion of 1500 mg or more.

Benzodiazepines are widely used for their sedative and tranquillizing properties. A wide variety is manufactured, varying mainly in terms of their length of therapeutic action. Each has a chemical and a trade or proprietary name, which is often different in different parts of the world. Short-acting benzodiazepines include triazolam and midazolam; intermediate-acting drugs comprise oxazepam, temezepam, flunitrazepam, lorezepam etc.; and the longer-acting group includes compounds such as flurazepam, nitrazepam, diazepam, chlordiazepoxide etc.

Blood levels in fatal cases vary greatly, but the following is a guide to severe and possibly lethal toxicity: nitrazepam 5–10 mg/L, diazepam 5–18 mg/L, chlordiazepoxide more than 20 mg/L.

The phenothiazines are a group of major tranquillizing psychoactive drugs (often termed neuroleptic drugs), which includes chlormethiazole, chlorpromazine (Largactil), haloperidol (butyrophenone), fluphenazine, promazine, trifluoroperazine and prochlorperazine. Autopsy appearances in deaths

from these substances are essentially negative, and analysis of body fluids is the only practical way – in conjunction with the circumstantial evidence – of proving the cause of death. Most deaths are thought to be due to abrupt cardiac dysrhythmias, convulsions or respiratory depression. A rare side-effect of many of these drugs is the neuroleptic malignant syndrome, which comprises hyperthermia, sweating, decreased consciousness and cardiovascular symptoms, which may lead to death. Combination of these drugs with alcohol and other hypnotics or sedatives markedly enhances their dangers.

The monoamine oxidase inhibitors (MAOIs) are well known to have specific dangers and should not be taken with a wide range of drugs (morphine, antihistamines, adrenaline, amphetamines etc.) or some foods containing tyramine (cheeses, yeast extracts, red wine, beans etc.), as the ensuing sympathomimetic effects may significantly raise the blood pressure and cause a cerebral haemorrhage. Drugs of this type include tranylcypromine, isocarboxazid and phenelzine. A reversible MAOI, moclobemide, is said to have fewer interactions with either tyramine or the drugs noted above.

BARBITURATES

Although it has already been mentioned that action by doctors and the introduction of pharmaceutical controls in many countries have led to the virtual outlawing of these drugs as hypnotics, they are still prescribed in many countries around the world, where they are consumed in large quantities and, as a result, they are a common form of drug dependence. These drugs are easily obtained on the illicit market. They are descriptively divided into long-acting, intermediate-acting and short-acting compounds. This division has an effect on the dosage that may be toxic and the blood levels that may be expected in fatal cases.

The short-acting barbiturates include the anaesthetics thiopentone, hexobarbitone, cyclobarbitone and secobarbital. Large doses of these drugs can cause death within about half an hour. The blood level found in fatal poisoning is about 17 mg/L (range 5–50 mg/L). The intermediate-acting drugs include amylobarbitone, pentobarbitone, allobarbitone and butobarbitone. The mean fatal level of this type of barbiturate is around 25 mg/L (range 10–70 mg/L. The

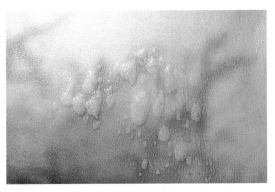

Figure 25.2 Blistering of the leg in a deeply comatose patient. Formerly called 'barbiturate blisters', they can be found in any condition leading to prolonged unconsciousness.

long-acting barbiturates, still used for the control of epilepsy, are drugs such as phenobarbitone and phenytoin. These have still higher therapeutic blood levels and levels in excess of 120 mg/L are required to cause death.

At autopsy, positive signs of fatal barbiturate overdoses include the presence of the remnants of coloured capsules in the stomach and erosions of the gastric mucosa, particularly when alkaline compounds such as amylobarbitone have been taken. There will commonly be general signs of marked congestion, with almost black lungs and cyanotic lividity due to the fatal, central respiratory failure. There may also be the so-called 'barbiturate blisters' on the dependent skin, most commonly on the thighs, backs of the arms and thorax. The blisters are due to oedema of the dependent skin as a result of poor venous return, which follows total immobility due to coma. These blisters are not specific to barbiturates, despite the name, and can be found in any drug-induced coma or, indeed, sometimes in a natural coma.

The simultaneous ingestion of alcohol or other hypnotic drugs greatly enhances the effects of barbiturates and any additive action, which may well result in respiratory as well as the cortical depression.

CHLORAL

Though an unfashionable drug in the modern pharmacopoeia, trichloracetaldehyde is still widely used in less sophisticated medical services, and patients can become addicted. Gastric ulceration and sometimes liver damage may follow the ingestion of chloral. An overdose of between 3 and 12 g may prove fatal, though analytical measurement is difficult due to rapid detoxification. Chronic alcoholics may be more susceptible to the toxic effects of chloral.

PHENACETIN

This analgesic has been abandoned in all but a few countries because of its toxic effects on the kidney. Phenacetin is converted to paracetamol in the liver and can have the same toxic effects on the liver as paracetamol. Phenacetin can also cause red cell haemolysis and methaemoglobinaemia.

LITHIUM

A number of medical negligence cases are brought against psychiatrists each year for failing to monitor lithium treatment in various psychiatric conditions. Lithium carbonate is thought to assist the uptake of noradrenaline by neurons, so reducing the availability of this neurotransmitter. It should never be used in pregnancy because of the increased risk of cardiac malformations in the fetus. Its toxic action on patients includes diarrhoea, vomiting, electrolyte disturbances, dysarthria and vertigo; polyuria and hyperosmolar coma may precede death. The choice of patient for this drug must be made with care and it is essential to choose patients with no previous renal or cardiovascular disease, and regular plasma lithium levels must be taken to ensure that they do not exceed 1.5 mmol/L, as the safety margin for this drug is small and levels of 2.0 mmol/L can lead to severe side-effects.

INSULIN

This therapeutic substance is one of the few that has been used repeatedly for homicide and is not infrequently used for suicide, usually amongst nurses and doctors who have access to large doses. However, unless an overdose of insulin is suspected, it is extremely difficult to diagnose. Insulin is an effective homicidal poison, even though modern methods of post-mortem assay now exist, as the complex investigations that are necessary to establish the diagnosis are unlikely to be launched unless there is some suspicion attached to what appears to be a natural death.

Insulin is, of course, a potent hypoglycaemic agent and, if severe lowering of the blood sugar persists for many hours, brain damage and death will occur. In massive doses, especially intravenously, death can take place within a very few hours. If death from insulin is suspected, whether suicide, homicide or accident, a search of the body must be made for recent needle marks, and the surrounding skin, subcutaneous tissue and underlying muscle must be excised and sent, unfixed, for assay. Blood samples should also be taken, as modern analytical methods can now distinguish between human, bovine and porcine insulin and can detect adjuvants such as zinc, which may assist in tracing the origin of any extrinsic insulin.

Post-mortem samples should be taken as soon as possible after death and the plasma immediately separated from the cells and then kept deep-frozen until analysis. Post-mortem blood glucose levels are generally unhelpful in confirming hypoglycaemia, but vitreous humour glucose levels may be more useful.

Oral hypoglycaemic agents, such as the sulphonylureas and biguanides, may be taken in overdose, either suicidally or accidentally, and produce hypoglycaemia, hyperkalaemia and acidosis.

Chapter twenty-six

Corrosive and Metallic Poisons

Corrosive poisons	Arsenic	Lead
Oxalic acid	Antimony	Thallium
Heavy-metal poisoning	Mercury	Iron

Corrosive and metallic poisons used to be quite common in Westernized countries as both suicidal and homicidal agents. Severe restrictions on their availability and the increasing ease with which these poisons are detected have markedly limited their use. However, in other parts of the world they are still used sufficiently frequently to ensure their continued inclusion in a forensic textbook. It is also important to remember these poisons whenever a death occurs, as lack of recent experience of them may lead the death investigator or the pathologist to assume that this type of poisoning could not happen in their country and so incorrectly dismiss it as a possibility.

CORROSIVE POISONS

Corrosive substances are used as suicidal poisons and for homicide and assaults in the form of 'acid bombs'; they are also used as agents of torture (see Chapter 21).

Corrosives irritate, necrose or destroy any surface with which they come into contact. These actions are a function of both the concentration of the substance and the length of time for which it acts, so rapid dilution and washing will greatly reduce the damage, whether internally or externally. If used in a very concentrated form, the damage is almost instantaneous and is likely to be very severe.

The action of any corrosive substance is a surface phenomenon, whether on the skin or the respiratory or gastrointestinal mucosa, but continued contact will enable the corrosion to penetrate deeply, so perforation of internal structures such as the oesophagus or stomach may occur with prolonged exposure.

There is often spillage of the corrosive agent on the exterior of the body, and the patterns of skin injury can help to reconstruct the way in which the substance was taken or applied. For example, a person swallowing acid or alkali from a cup whilst standing or sitting usually has overflow marks around the corners of the mouth and dribbles that run down the chin, neck and perhaps chest. If they were lying down or had immediately fallen back, the trickle marks are likely to be down the side of the face, cheeks and on to the side of the neck. Coughing and spluttering may project the poison on to the hands, clothing or nearby objects – the fingers are often held to the mouth and also become corroded. Deliberate splashing with acid will result in areas or spots of injury and there may be vertical dribbles from the points of contact if the victim was standing. The patterns produced by accidental splashing will depend upon the position of the individual when splashed, and this information should be specifically sought from work colleagues and other witnesses.

Internally, oesophageal and gastric damage is to be expected if the substance is swallowed, and there may also be overflow into the glottis and larynx, with

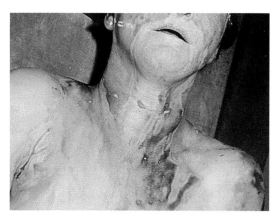

Figure 26.1 Suicidal ingestion of a corrosive substance (Lysol). Spillage around the mouth has run down the neck and onto the chest.

aspiration into the trachea and bronchi, which may cause extensive damage. Lung damage and broncho-pneumonia are common sequelae if the victim survives the acute phase. Vomiting is an additional risk as acid or alkali already swallowed may be aspirated into the larynx during uncontrolled regurgitation.

If victims survive, they may need surgical repair of acute perforations and, at a later stage, treatment for stenosis caused by scarring of the oesophagus, pharynx and stomach.

The common corrosives include:

- acids – such as the strong mineral acids (sulphuric, nitric and hydrochloric) and the organic acids like acetic, formic and oxalic;
- alkalis – such as sodium hydroxide (caustic soda or 'lye'), potassium hydroxide, calcium hydroxide (lime) and ammonium hydroxide;
- miscellaneous substances – such as lysol (phenol or carbolic), salts of heavy metals, household bleaches and strong detergents; many metal polishes, household cleaners and some toilet cleaners containing sodium hypochlorite and sodium acid sulphate are also corrosive.

The symptoms are obvious and immediate, with pain at the sites of exposure, usually the mouth and on the skin, difficulty in swallowing, chest pain, abdominal pain, vomiting, difficulty in breathing, choking. If the amount ingested is significant, there will be signs of shock, with collapse, a weak and rapid pulse, hypotension and possibly death, even if treatment is available straightaway.

At autopsy, the lips, face and any other affected skin are likely to be discoloured and corroded, but this will depend upon the amount, type and concentration of the corrosive. Corrosion may extend for a variable distance down into the pharynx, oesophagus and stomach and may even extend into the small intestine, depending upon the volume swallowed. Damage in the air passages has already been mentioned.

Acids tend to corrode and thicken the mucosa, whereas alkalis turn the lining into a slimy, soft pulp. Perforation of the oesophagus or stomach is most common with sulphuric, hydrochloric or hydrofluoric acids, but the danger exists with all corrosives when washing out with a stomach tube.

Oxalic acid

Although not as corrosive as the mineral acids, oxalic acid and potassium quadroxalate are very toxic, death often occurring within a hour or so if the solid or concentrated solution is taken. They are used extensively as stain removers and in many other trades and industries.

Oxalic acid crystals look like the innocuous magnesium sulphate (Epsom salts) and have been ingested in mistake for it. Oxalic acid is both locally corrosive and acts as a systemic poison. Dilute solutions may cause minimal damage to the skin and mucosal surfaces but may still prove fatal. When swallowed, the mucosa of the mouth and oesophagus is bleached, though the whiteness can be streaked with red haemorrhage. The stomach contains black, altered blood, and calcium oxalate crystals can sometimes be seen adherent to the ulcerated mucosa. The systemic effect is mainly due to the well-known effect of oxalate on calcium (it is used *in vitro* to prevent clotting in blood samples). The body calcium is precipitated as insoluble calcium oxalate, leading to abnormalities of muscle function from hypocalcaemia. Renal failure also occurs and in survivors of the acute phase of poisoning, necrosis of the proximal convoluted tubules may be seen. Calcium oxalate crystals may be seen microscopically in the kidney, although they are not the direct cause of the necrosis.

HEAVY-METAL POISONING

The history of forensic toxicology is closely linked to the use of certain metallic poisons as agents of homicide.

The literature of nineteenth-century European forensic medicine is full of notorious cases of murder by arsenic, antimony and mercury. Occasional cases still occur so all doctors should retain some index of suspicion, especially where atypical gastrointestinal symptoms exist and do not respond to treatment. There are very few instances of metallic poisoning from industrial exposure in the UK because of the awareness of the dangers and the supervision of the health and safety inspectors. However, toxic effects and deaths from metallic poisons are still common in regions where such occupational and environmental safeguards are less effective.

Arsenic

Arsenic is the twelfth most common element and is itself not poisonous; it is the compounds of arsenic, particularly arsenious oxide and the various arsenites of copper, sodium and potassium, that are toxic to humans. These compounds exert their effects by combining with the sulphydryl groups of mitochondrial enzymes and so prevent cellular respiration. Vascular endothelium appears to be particularly susceptible to the toxic effects of arsenic. Arsenical substances are widely used in industry and agriculture but are now seldom, if ever, used in conventional medicine. Of historical interest is the fact that many former editions of this book needed to list a number of sources of pharmacological arsenic. Once ingested, arsenic is stored for long periods in certain tissues and remains permanently in hair, skin and nails (sulphur-containing keratin) until they are shed.

Poisoning is rare and may be suicidal or homicidal, but accidental and environmental causes are more likely. The signs and symptoms of arsenical poisoning have so often been mistaken for a natural intestinal disease that some account must be offered. Acute and chronic poisoning must be considered separately, as there are marked differences between a single ingestion of a large dose, as in most suicides, and accidental or environmental poisoning, where there is more likely to be the insidious onset of chronic toxicity from repeated small doses.

In acute poisoning, if sufficient chemical is ingested, there may be initial burning in the mouth and then, after an interval, signs of intense gastroenteritis develop: abdominal pain, nausea, burning regurgitation and vomiting. Diarrhoea ensues and this, together with the sickness, leads to prostration, mainly from dehydration and electrolyte imbalance. The faeces soon become watery and often blood streaked. Thirst, oliguria, cramps, collapse and perhaps convulsions lead to cardiovascular failure and death, sometimes within hours if the dose is large, though survival can last for several days. In massive dosage, death may occur before these signs have time to appear.

In chronic poisoning, a classic state of ill-health develops, which has often been attributed, incorrectly, to some systemic natural illness. Loss of appetite, mild nausea, some vomiting, jaundice, loss of weight and anaemia are relatively non-specific symptoms, which – especially in the days when ancillary investigations were minimal – have been accepted as being incapable of further diagnosis or treatment. More specific signs can be seen in the skin, where chronic arsenical poisoning causes hyperkeratosis of the palms of the hands and soles of the feet, a speckled pigmentation of the general skin surface (sometimes described as a 'raindrop' appearance with patches of pale leucoplakia), loss of hair, brittle nails and a peripheral neuritis with itching, tingling and paraesthesia of the extremities, sometimes with painful swelling (erythromelalgia).

The fatal dose is variable, but 200–300 mg of arsenious oxide are likely to be needed for acute fatal toxicity. At autopsy, little may be found in acute deaths apart from a haemorrhagic gastritis. The stomach mucosa has been likened to red velvet, due to the bleeding along the top ridges of the mucosal folds, which are also oedematous. Subendocardial bleeding may be seen in the left ventricle, though this is not specific to arsenic and can be seen in any death when there has been a precipitous drop in blood pressure due to 'shock'.

In chronic poisoning, the autopsy will reveal a series of non-specific signs – wasting, atrophy and dehydration together with skin thickening, hair loss and puffiness of the face – may be found and degenerative changes can be identified in liver, myocardium and kidneys. There is no good evidence for the long-standing claim that people dying of chronic arsenic poisoning resist post-mortem decomposition far longer than normal, apart from the possibility that dehydration sometimes inhibits the rapid onset of moist putrefaction.

Internally, the stomach may show a chronic gastritis with excess mucus and patchy mucosal erosion. The gut may reveal a non-specific mixed oedema and enteritis or it may appear quite normal, apart from a copious 'rice-water' content. The liver may suffer fatty degeneration or even necrosis, usually at the periphery of the lobules. Renal tubular damage and sometimes myocardial necrosis can occur.

In any suspected arsenical poisoning, samples of hair, nails, blood, urine, faeces and any vomit should be collected from live subjects, supplemented by stomach and contents, intestinal contents, liver, kidneys and bile from autopsies. The samples should be submitted to an expert toxicologist for analysis, as the days of do-it-yourself meddling with the Marsh, Reinsch and Gutzeit tests are now strictly part of medical history.

The ubiquitous nature of arsenic means that if a body is being exhumed because of possible arsenical poisoning, control samples of soil from the grave and of the grave water should be taken so that the role of natural exposure to arsenic after burial can be considered.

It was formerly thought that it took a week or two for ingested arsenic to appear in the keratinized tissues such as hair and nails, but the more sensitive analytical techniques now used have shown that the metal can appear there within hours. The test for determining when the arsenic was administered, by measuring the concentration in different parts of the hair shaft at varying distances from the growing root, is still a useful tool for establishing chronicity of exposure. The metal can remain in keratinized tissues for several years after administration of arsenic has ceased.

Antimony

Antimony is quite similar to arsenic, both in symptomatology and fatal dosage. The usual compound encountered in suicide, accident and the very rare homicide is antimony potassium tartrate, often called 'tartar emetic'. Poisoning of numbers of people in the same incident has taken place following the absorption of antimony from the enamel lining of cooking utensils. Although 150 mg has proved fatal, it is more common for there to be a full recovery from vastly greater doses; indeed, 150 mg used to be the intravenous dosage when antimony was used in the treatment of bilharzia.

Mercury

Mercury is usually an industrial or environmental poison. Although historically some deaths occurred from its use in medicine, mercurial diuretics and antiseptics are now almost a thing of the past.

Acute poisoning resembles that of arsenic and antimony: gastrointestinal symptoms are common, but there are also excessive salivation and signs of renal failure. Chronic mercury poisoning is almost wholly industrial in nature and the clinical hallmarks are gingivitis, loose teeth, salivation, black gums, mandibular necrosis, peripheral neuritis, encephalopathy and renal failure.

Lead

Lead poisoning is also now an industrial and environmental problem, especially since the last forensic aspects of lead-induced criminal abortions have passed into history.

Thallium

Thallium has been used homicidally several times in recent years, most notably by Graham Young in Britain in 1971, when two victims died and others narrowly avoided death. This case was forensically unique in that it was probably the first murder in which the poison was detected posthumously in the ashes of a cremated victim. Thallium is also unusual in being detectable radiologically in the intestine and liver.

Thallium is used as a rat poison and is widely employed in industry, especially for optical glass. It is no longer used medically to remove hair in skin diseases because of its toxicity. Hair loss is a major sign of poisoning and begins 1 or 2 weeks after oral administration. The other common symptoms of abdominal pain and vomiting characterize acute poisoning. In succeeding days and weeks, muscle pains, peripheral neuritis, confusion, sleep disturbances and psychiatric symptoms appear. At autopsy, widespread, but nonspecific, degeneration in the heart, liver, kidneys, brain and other organs is discovered.

Iron

Iron is best known in toxicology as an acute poison in children who have eaten the attractive-looking tablets of ferrous sulphate that had been prescribed for their mothers to treat anaemia. Death has occurred in small infants with as few as three to five tablets, gastrointestinal symptoms occurring soon after ingestion. There may be a temporary respite in symptoms, then a relapse, which is sometimes fatal due to liver damage and acidosis from the release of free iron into the circulation as a result of overloading the transferrin system, which normally binds excess iron to protein.

Chapter twenty-seven

Agrochemical Poisons

Pesticides and insecticides
Herbicides (weed killers)

Agrochemicals are important because they are used in such vast quantities in most parts of the world. These chemicals include pesticides and herbicides, which have greatly increased food yields but have brought their own dangers. They are particularly common and therefore particularly dangerous in rural and agricultural communities. Worldwide, there are millions of admissions to hospital and more than 250 000 deaths each year as a result of the ingestion of agrochemicals. Some are suicidal, a few homicidal, but most are the result of either accidental or environmental exposure. In the UK, over 40 per cent of suspected childhood poisonings are related to the ingestion of rodenticides.

PESTICIDES AND INSECTICIDES

First amongst this group are the organophosphate compounds, which kill insect pests by inhibiting choline esterase enzymes, thus preventing the breakdown of acetylcholine. One of the most toxic is parathion, though others such as malathion, dithion, demeton, octamethylpyrophosphamide (OMPA), hexaethyltetraphosphate (HETP) and tetraethylpyrophosphate (TEPP) are also poisonous. These and similar compounds have caused thousands of deaths, especially in South-East Asia, either by direct absorption or by contamination of foodstuffs with insecticides during storage or transit.

The organophosphates are sprayed in liquid form in a kerosene base or used as dusting powders. They can be absorbed through the intact skin, by inhalation or orally. Toxic effects begin when the choline esterase level drops below about 30 per cent of normal. With large doses, death may be very rapid; otherwise, nausea, vomiting, blurred vision, sweating, colic, contracted pupils and fits may precede death.

The organo-chlorine compounds include lindane, dieldrin and dicophane (DDT). They are soluble in body fat and are not nearly as toxic as the organophosphate compounds; indeed, fatalities are rare, though contaminated grain has caused extensive harm. Their disadvantage is that they get into the food chain and cause widespread harmful effects on wildlife; this is why the parathion-type substances were developed, as they are far less stable than DDT-like compounds.

HERBICIDES (WEED KILLERS)

The dipyridyl herbicides are also used in great quantities in many countries. The best known is paraquat, marketed to the trade as a liquid concentrate under the trade name Gramoxone and as a much weaker granular form for garden and horticultural use, as Weedol. Gramoxone is extremely toxic and one swallowed mouthful is commonly fatal unless immediate energetic treatment is undertaken. Most fatalities are suicidal, but quite a number of accidental poisonings occur, usually because the liquid is mistaken for a drink. In some countries, including the Republic of Ireland, it is a criminal offence to remove Gramoxone from its original marked container into any other receptacle, because of this risk of accidental poisoning.

Paraquat is corrosive, causing a burning sensation in the mouth and pharynx, with ulceration of the mucosa, but the grave effects are upon the liver, kidneys and lungs. Hepato-renal failure may occur within the first few days, with a centrilobular necrosis and tubular damage. If the victim survives for longer than a week, lung damage is common, with what is essentially the adult respiratory distress syndrome developing. A hyaline membrane forms and the alveoli fill with pneumocytes, which lead to pulmonary fibrosis if the patient lives for a few weeks. Diquat is a similar herbicide.

Chapter twenty-eight

Gaseous Poisons

| Carbon monoxide | Carbon dioxide | Ammonia | Cyanogen gas and cyanides |

A number of unrelated poisons are in gaseous form. Though there are many gaseous poisons in existence, especially in an industrial environment, only a few are seen frequently in forensic practice.

CARBON MONOXIDE

In many urbanized countries, 'coal gas' or 'town gas' used to be easily available in almost every home and, as it contained between 7 per cent and 20 per cent carbon monoxide (CO), it was a potent poison and was commonly used as a method of suicide, it also caused many accidental deaths. When natural gas became generally available, especially throughout Europe and North America, the number of deaths due to poisoning by CO was drastically reduced.

The change in house gas supply has not eliminated CO poisoning, and other sources of the gas have simply become more prominent. The exhaust gas from petrol engines (unless fitted with a modern catalytic converter) contains between 4 and 8 per cent CO; diesel engines produce less. In a common suicidal sequence, the victim either sits in the car in a closed garage with the engine running or leads a pipe from the exhaust through the window of the car.

The other common causes of CO poisoning, almost always accidental, are faulty gas appliances and heating systems. When any hydrocarbon fuel is burned in oxygen (O_2 – air), it will be completely converted into

carbon dioxide (CO_2) and water only if there is an adequate O_2 (air) supply. If air is restricted, CO will be formed instead of CO_2. This may occur in gas water heaters, boilers, fires, cookers etc. and in central heating units fuelled by coal, coke, butane, propane or oil. Faulty adjustment, insufficient ventilation and blocked chimneys and flues may lead to this danger. Such faulty appliances can insidiously kill whole families as they sleep in a house or caravan.

The other major source of CO is a fire in a house or building, where burning timber, furniture and fabrics can produce large volumes of the gas, together with other toxic gases, which kill far more people than actual burns. Other sources of CO are in industry, where huge volumes are produced and used in steel-works etc.

CO is a heavy, colourless gas, odourless when pure, but often contaminated by impurities, which have a smell. Its poisonous qualities are due to its great affinity for haemoglobin, as it has a combining power some 250 times greater than O_2. This means that even small concentrations of CO can displace O_2 from the red blood cells and progressively diminish the ability of the blood to transport O_2 to the tissues. Strong concentrations of CO, such as a leak from a laboratory cylinder, can kill within a few moments. Exercise (causing faster breathing) and the quicker respirations of children can hasten the absorption of a fatal level of CO.

There is great variation in personal susceptibility and in the speed with which saturation takes place. Levels of carboxyhaemoglobin saturation above 50–60 per cent are likely to be fatal in healthy adults, whereas old people and those with pulmonary or cardiac disease may well die at much lower levels, even down to 25 per cent saturation. The individual sensitivity of different people is well illustrated by multiple deaths in the same room, where bodies lying side by side may have markedly different saturation levels.

The clinical symptoms of CO poisoning are stealthy and progressive so that victims may not notice anything, except a headache, until they lapse into coma and die. Many cigarette smokers tolerate levels of up to 10–15 per cent without symptoms. At up to about 30 per cent saturation of the haemoglobin in fit adults, there may simply be headache and slight nausea; this is very likely to be associated with lack of concentration and even a slight 'drunkenness', which may be mistaken for alcohol, especially if driving skills are impaired.

At from 30 to 40 per cent saturation, nausea, possibly vomiting, faintness, loss of visual acuity, weakness and a slide towards stupor and coma begin. Over 40–50 per cent, sickness, weakness, incoordination, convulsions and coma will progress towards cardiorespiratory failure and death. Some fit young adults may reach 70 per cent saturation or more before dying. It must be emphasized that these figures are very variable, depending on age, fitness and personal susceptibility.

The stability of carboxyhaemoglobin makes it a cumulative poison, and the blood will continue to absorb the gas from the lungs if it is present in the inspired air, so that remarkably small concentrations of inspired CO may eventually prove fatal. Within 2–3 hours, even 0.1 per cent CO in the atmosphere may result in 55–60 per cent saturation. Within 20 minutes, 1 per cent CO can cause unconsciousness, and the air in a single garage with a 2-litre car engine running can reach a lethal level within 5 minutes.

The external signs of CO poisoning, apart from the symptoms, are a pink coloration of the skin, usually described as 'cherry-pink'. The nail beds and lips may also show this characteristic colour, but this may not be obvious in the living until high saturations are reached. In the hypostatic areas of the dead body, the pink coloration is usually obvious, but exceptions may be found in the old or anaemic, in whom reduction in haemoglobin content reduces the intensity of the coloration.

Internally, all the organs are pink in colour due to carboxyhaemoglobin and carboxymyoglobin. Pulmonary oedema is common but there are no specific organ changes, except in the brain of individuals who have survived for a time following an episode of CO poisoning, in which case there may be bilateral cystic

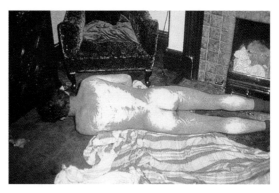

Figure 28.1 Cherry-pink hypostasis of carbon monoxide poisoning.

degeneration of the basal ganglia. Individuals with long-term survival following significant exposure may have a parkinsonian syndrome or may develop even worse neurological states. Long-term psychological damage may also be caused and this, too, is associated with the profound cerebral hypoxia of CO poisoning.

Confirmation of CO poisoning in both the living and dead depends upon analysis of blood.

CARBON DIOXIDE

CO_2 is a relatively inert gas and, unlike the monoxide, is neither directly poisonous nor is it a cumulative poison. However, it can still kill, because it is an irrespirable gas. Three per cent in the atmosphere will cause headache, drowsiness, giddiness and loss of muscle power.

Sources of CO_2 are often industrial as it is used very widely in the manufacture of many products. In anaesthesia, deaths have occurred when an O_2 cylinder has become empty whilst connected to a functioning CO_2 cylinder, so that the patient has received only CO_2.

Vagrants 'sleeping rough' near lime kilns are said to have died due to this heavier-than-air gas creeping over them during the night. Most modern fatalities are associated with wells, deep shafts and farming exposure. In chalk rock, CO_2 can accumulate in deep holes and this has caused deaths of workmen and, in one instance, of a doctor who descended a well to give help. On farms, the tall grain silos can fill with CO_2 produced by the respiration of the seed; the CO_2 sinks to the bottom and when workers enter through a hatch to clear blockages in the delivery chutes, they may be rapidly overcome.

An unexplained feature of CO_2 is the speed of its toxicity on many occasions. Pure asphyxia should take several minutes and be associated with cyanosis and congestion, but CO_2 deaths can be very rapid and there are seldom any 'asphyxial signs'. It is presumed that this is due to some vasovagal reflex causing cardiac arrest, triggered by a chemoreceptor stimulus.

The minimum fatal concentration of CO_2 is said to be 25–30 per cent, the high concentrations causing sudden death being 60–80 per cent.

AMMONIA

Ammonia gas is an uncommon poison outside industry. It was formerly used extensively in refrigeration but has been largely replaced by more inert fluids. Ammonia is occasionally used criminally for aiding assaults and robberies by being thrown in the face, and this is sometimes also done in attempts to blind or scar. In gaseous form, escapes in factories may cause severe lung symptoms, choking and coughing, and pulmonary oedema may be followed by bronchopneumonia.

CYANOGEN GAS AND CYANIDES

Hydrogen cyanide (HCN) is a gas; hydrocyanic acid (prussic acid) is a solution of HCN in water, either 2 per cent or 4 per cent, the latter being called Scheele's acid. Salts of cyanide, usually sodium and potassium, are white solids. Cyanides are extremely poisonous, their action depending upon the inhibition of the respiratory enzyme cytochrome oxidase, thus preventing the utilization of O_2 by tissue cells.

Cyanides are used in industry for a wide variety of processes, as well as in photography, electroplating and laboratory techniques. They are also used as vermin killers and, regrettably, are still in use as weapons of war. Fumigation of trees, fruit and ships is common and accounts for a number of accidental deaths. Chemists and laboratory workers are sometimes overcome by HCN generated by cyanides being poured into sinks and drains that already contain acid. Suicide by cyanide

is not uncommon, especially amongst laboratory staff who have easy access to the substances. In one survey of cyanide deaths, 70 per cent were found to be self-administered. The use of cyanide in homicides is not common, but it has been deliberately substituted for drugs of dependence and it has been used to contaminate medicinal drugs for sale in pharmacies and, in the notorious Jonesville tragedy in Guyana, 900 people died of cyanide poisoning instigated by the 'Reverend' Jim Jones.

Cyanide is only poisonous as free cyanide and therefore swallowed salts need to encounter either water or gastric acid before liberating HCN, a process which takes only a few seconds. The fatal dose of cyanide, in the form of a salt, is only 150–300 mg, which allows it to be concealed as 'suicide pills' in rings or hollow teeth. However, recovery has been recorded with far larger doses of up to 2.4 g of potassium cyanide.

Symptoms and death are often very rapid but not necessarily so – treatment has saved many victims of cyanide ingestion. Though some literally 'drop dead' within seconds, many linger for 15–20 minutes, even after substantial doses, depending upon the speed of absorption.

The blood remains pink, due to failure of uptake of O_2 by the tissues. The skin, especially after death, may be a brick-red colour, particularly in the dependent hypostasis. This may be confused with CO poisoning, though cyanide usually gives a darker, sometimes purplish hue, whereas CO has a pinker colour.

Cyanides have a characteristic smell, but up to 80 per cent of the general population have a congenital inability to detect the odour of bitter almonds. Those who cannot detect the smell of cyanide may instead report a sudden onset of a severe headache due to the cerebral vasodilatation caused by this chemical. At autopsy, great care must be taken to reduce the exposure of individuals in the mortuary to a minimum, and breathing hoods should be worn. The organs will be congested and bright or dark red. If cyanide has been swallowed, the oesophagus and stomach lining will be deep red or black, especially along the rugal folds, due to erosion and haemorrhage, and the smell of cyanide may be most obvious when the stomach is opened.

Chapter twenty-nine

Miscellaneous Poisons

Strychnine   Gasoline and kerosene   Nicotine

Halogenated hydrocarbons   The glycols

STRYCHNINE

Strychnine is an alkaloid prepared from the seeds of the *Nux vomica* tree. In pure form it is a colourless crystal and has a notable extremely bitter taste. It is one of the cruellest poisons in existence as it causes excruciating agony to any form of animal life whilst not affecting consciousness. Used to kill 'pests', from earthworms to dogs, there is no justification for its continued use or even manufacture, as it no longer has any place in medical treatment and its use in the barbaric killing of animals is quite unjustifiable.

A fatal dose may be as little as 30–60 mg, though, as usual, there is great individual variation. Its major effect is upon the muscles, as twitching begins soon after absorption, deepening into muscle spasms, then developing into convulsions. Opisthotonus and risus sardonicus – the grin induced by the contracted facial muscles – indicate the widespread muscle stimulation.

Through stimulation of the central nervous system, especially the spinal reflexes, muscles go into tetanic spasms and tetanus may be the differential diagnosis where no history is available. The spasms may tear muscles from their ligaments and tendons by the gross contractions; all the while, the maintenance of consciousness allows the appreciation of the excruciating pain. Episodes of convulsive muscle spasm are triggered by minimal stimulation, and exhaustion aided by respiratory failure due to spasm and loss of

function in the intercostal and diaphragmatic muscles leads to death.

There are no specific features at autopsy, apart from haemorrhage into traumatized muscle, and the tendon insertions, routine retention of samples of gastric contents, blood and urine will reveal strychnine on toxicological analysis.

HALOGENATED HYDROCARBONS

This group comprises a number of compounds in which part of the aliphatic chain is replaced by one or more halogen atoms. The resulting substances are in widespread used in industry, refrigeration, dry cleaning and medicine, one of the latter being Trilene anaesthetic (tri-chlorethylene). All of these chemicals are active fat solvents and have deleterious effects on the liver, causing hepatic cell damage that may proceed to necrosis.

Though most exposure is accidental, self-administration as a form of addiction may also be seen and this may lead to anaesthetists inhaling their own agents or to abuse of solvents or other halogenated compounds on the streets. Absorption may be from ingestion, inhalation or even skin contact, where the body surface may suffer from the strong fat-solvent action of these substances.

Methylene chloride is widely used in refrigeration and many deaths and toxic states have occurred from leakage from refrigeration plants. Chronic exposure may lead to cerebellar signs, with staggering gait, dizziness, vertigo and visual disturbances. Methyl bromide is used in fire extinguishers and as an insecticide. It can blister skin and mucous membranes. Exposure may lead to muscular incoordination, ataxia and muscle twitching. Renal tubular necrosis may also develop.

Carbon tetrachloride used to be available as a domestic dry-cleaning agent (Thawpit) and a fire extinguisher (Pyrene) as well as commercial solvent. It is a liver poison, but not as dangerous in this respect as tetrachlorethane. Excessive domestic use of the stain remover could lead to anaesthesia and it could also become addictive. Death can occur, especially if drunk by children. When sprayed on a burning surface as a fire extinguisher, carbon tetrachloride could be converted to the even more toxic gas phosgene.

Tetrachlorethane is nine times as toxic as carbon tetrachloride. It is also a solvent and plasticizer used for films, artificial pearls etc. Its original use as a solvent for cellulose in aircraft 'dope' was abandoned early in the twentieth century when jaundice and deaths occurred in the factory workers. Liver necrosis may be accompanied by a polyneuritis affecting the extremities of the limbs.

GASOLINE AND KEROSENE

Petrol and paraffin, alternative names for these fuels, can cause coma and death within a few minutes if swallowed or inhaled in high concentration. If drunk, they may also be coughed or vomited into the air passages, where they spread widely and rapidly due to their low surface tension, damaging surfactant and precipitating bronchopneumonia if the victim survives the initial direct toxic effects.

THE GLYCOLS

Used as industrial solvents and anti-freeze agents for motor engines, the glycols are sometimes misused, either for suicide or, more often, as a cheap substitute for alcoholic drinks. Accidental ingestion usually occurs when they have been put into an unlabelled soft-drink bottle. Of the several glycols – dioxan (diethylene dioxide), ethylene chlorhydrin etc. – ethylene glycol is most toxic and most widely available. If drunk in excess of about 100–200 mL, it is likely to be fatal unless energetic treatment such as renal dialysis is instituted.

Though symptoms resembling mild drunkenness appear at first, death may supervene within a day or so because part of the metabolic pathway converts glycol through formic acid to oxalic acid. Renal failure occurs, with fan-shaped crystals of calcium oxalate in the kidney tubules and interstitial tissues. Liver damage may also occur.

NICOTINE

Though homicides have been committed with nicotine, most fatal poisonings are accidental, usually from insecticides, some of which may be almost pure nicotine. The poison can be absorbed by mouth, by inhalation or through the skin and death has resulted from the ingestion or application of as little as 40 mg. Even tobacco leaves wrapped around sweaty skin during smuggling have caused serious toxic effects, as have the tar and remnants of pipe and cigarette smoking to children.

Nicotine paralyses muscles and usually kills by depressing the respiratory musculature, as well as producing sweating, dizziness, fainting and convulsions.

Guidelines for an Autopsy and Exhumation

Guidelines for a medico-legal autopsy
The autopsy

GUIDELINES FOR A MEDICO-LEGAL AUTOPSY

1 Where the death is definitely due to crime or if there is a possibility of crime (a suspicious death), the doctor should attend the scene (locus) before the body is moved in order to gain an understanding of the surroundings, blood distribution in relation to the body etc. Notes of attendance, of people present and of the observations should be made. Photographs should be taken of the scene in general, of the body in particular and of any other significant features; these are usually taken by the police.

2 The identity of the body should be confirmed to the doctor by a relative or by a police officer or other legal officer who either knows the deceased personally or who has had the body positively identified to them by a relative or by some other means (e.g. fingerprints).

3 If the remains are mummified, skeletalized, decomposed, burnt or otherwise disfigured to a point at which visual identification is impossible or uncertain, or if the identity is unknown, other methods of establishing the identity of the remains must be used, but the autopsy cannot be delayed while this is done.

4 In a suspicious death, if there can be no direct identification of the body, a police officer must confirm directly to the doctor that the body or the remains presented for autopsy are those that are the focus of the police inquiry.

5 In a suspicious death, the body should be examined with the clothing in place so that defects caused by trauma that may have damaged the body (stabs wounds, gunshot injuries etc.) can be identified. When removed, the clothing must be retained in new, clean bags that are sealed and carefully labelled for later forensic science examination.

6 In suspicious deaths or if there are any unusual features, the body should be photographed clothed and then unclothed and then any injuries or other abnormalities should be photographed in closer detail.

7 X-rays are advisable in victims of gunshot wounds and explosions and where there is a possibility of retained metal fragments, and are mandatory in all suspicious deaths in children.

8 The surface of the body should be examined for the presence of trace evidence: fibres, hair, blood, saliva, semen etc. This examination may be performed by police officers or by forensic scientists, often with the assistance of the pathologist. Where samples are to be removed from the body itself as opposed to the surface of the body – fingernail clippings, head and pubic hair, anal and genital swabs – these should be taken by the pathologist.

9 Forensic scientists may also wish to examine the body using specialist techniques, and the pathologist must be aware of their needs and allow them access at appropriate times.

10 Careful documentation of the external features of injuries or abnormalities, their position, size, shape and type, is often the most important aspect of a forensic examination and often has much greater value in understanding and in reconstructing the circumstances of injury than the internal dissection of any wound tracks or of damaged internal organs. Patience is required to perform this examination with care and this part of an examination should not be rushed.

11 The internal examination must fulfil two requirements: to identify and document injuries and to identify and document natural disease. The former may involve the examination of wound tracks caused by knives, bullets or other penetrating objects. It may also involve determining the extent and depth of bruising on the body by reflecting the skin from all of the body surfaces and identifying and describing areas of trauma to the internal organs.

12 A complete internal examination of all three body cavities, with dissection of all of the body organs, must be performed to identify any underlying natural disease.

13 Samples of blood (for blood grouping, DNA analysis, toxicology) and urine (for toxicology) will be routinely requested by the police. Blood should be collected from a large limb vein, preferably the femoral vein, and urine should be collected, preferably using a clean syringe, through the fundus of the bladder. All samples should be collected into clean containers, which are sealed and labelled in the presence of the pathologist. Care must be taken to ensure that the correct preservative is added; if in doubt, ask a forensic scientist for advice.

14 When poisoning is suspected, other samples, including stomach contents, intestinal contents, samples of organs including liver, kidney, lung and brain, may be requested. The storage, preservation and handling of these specimens will depend upon the suspected poison. Specialist advice must be obtained or the samples may be useless.

15 Tissue samples should be retained in formalin for microscopic examination. If there is any doubt, whole organs – brain and heart in particular – should be retained for specialist examination.

16 In all of these aspects of the examination, careful notes must be kept and augmented by drawings and diagrams if necessary. These notes, drawings and diagrams will form the basis for the report.

THE AUTOPSY

More detailed instructions for the internal examination are contained within a number of books in the 'Recommended reading' list at the end of the book. A short summary of the basic techniques is given below.

1 An incision is made from the larynx to the pubis. The upper margin may be extended on each side of the neck to form a 'Y' incision. The extra exposure this brings is useful in cases of neck injury or in children.

2 The skin on the front of the chest and abdomen is reflected laterally and the anterior abdominal wall is opened, taking care not to damage the intestines. The intestines are removed by cutting through the third part of the duodenum as it emerges from the retroperitoneum and then dissecting the small and large bowel from the mesentery.

3 The ribs are sawn through in a line from the lateral costal margin to the inner clavicle and the front of the chest is removed.

4 The tongue and pharynx are mobilized by passing a knife around the floor of the mouth close to the mandible. These are then removed downward as the neck structures are dissected off the cervical spine.

5 The axillary vessels are divided at the clavicles, and the oesophagus and the aorta are dissected from the thoracic spine as the tongue continues to be pulled forwards and downwards.

6 The lateral and posterior attachments of the diaphragm are cut through close to the chest cavity wall and then the aorta is dissected off the lower thoracic and lumbar spine.

7 Finally, the iliac vessels and the ureters can be bisected at the level of the pelvic rim and the organs will then be free of the body and can be taken to a table for dissection.

8 The pelvic organs are examined *in situ* or they can be removed from the pelvis for examination.

9 The scalp is incised coronally and the flaps reflected forwards and backwards. The skull-cap is carefully sawn through and removed, leaving the dura intact. This is then incised and the brain removed by gentle traction of the frontal lobes while cutting through the cranial nerves, the tentorium and the upper spinal cord.

10 The organs are dissected in a good light with adequate water to maintain an essentially blood-free area. Although every pathologist has his or her own order of dissection, a novice would do well to stick to the following order so that nothing is omitted: tongue, carotid arteries, oesophagus, larynx, trachea, thyroid, lungs, great vessels, heart, stomach, intestines, adrenals, kidneys, spleen, pancreas, gall

bladder and bile ducts, liver, bladder, uterus and ovaries or testes and finally the brain.

11 Samples should be taken for toxicology and histology as necessary.

12 Make detailed notes at the time of your examination and write your report as soon as possible, even if you cannot complete it because further tests are being performed.

13 All reports should include all of the positive findings and all of the relevant negative findings, because in court the absence of a comment may be taken to mean that it was not examined or specifically looked for and, if a hearing or trial is delayed for many months or years, it would not be credible to state that specific details of this examination can be remembered with clarity.

14 The conclusions should be concise and address all of the relevant issues concerning the death of the individual. A conclusion about the cause of death will be reached in most cases, but in some it is acceptable to give a differential list of causes from which the court may choose.

Preparation of the Reagent for the Kastle–Meyer Test

The following reagent is prepared:

130 mg phenolphthalein
1.3 g potassium hydroxide
100 mL distilled water

This is boiled until clear, then 20 g of powdered zinc are added. A few drops of this reagent are mixed with an equal volume of 20-vol. hydrogen peroxide. No colour should result, indicating that the reagents and glassware are not contaminated. The mixed reagent is then added to the filter paper or stain extract and an almost instant strong pink colour indicates the probability of blood being present. If benzidene is still used in your laboratory, a fresh 20 per cent solution of the powder in glacial acetic acid is added to an equal volume of peroxide before adding to the test material. An instant, intense deep-blue colour indicates positivity.

Recommended Reading

Autopsy procedures and anthropology
Forensic medicine and pathology

Medical ethics
Toxicology

Websites

AUTOPSY PROCEDURES AND ANTHROPOLOGY

Burton, J. and Rutty, G. (eds) 2001. *The Hospital Autopsy*, 2nd edition. London: Arnold.

Haglund, W.D. and Sorg, M.H. 1996. *Forensic Taphonomy*. Boca Raton, IL: CRC Press.

Krogman, W. and Iscan, M.Y. 1986. *The Skeleton in Forensic Medicine*, 2nd edition. Springfield, IL: Charles C Thomas.

Ludwig, J. 1979. *Current Methods in Autopsy Practice*, 2nd edition. Philadelphia: W.B. Saunders.

Trotter, M. and Gleser, G.C. 1958. A Re-evaluation of Estimation of Stature on Measurements of Stature Taken During Life and of Long Bones After Death. *American Journal of Physical Anthropology* **16: 79–123**.

Trotter, M. and Gleser, G.C. 1977. Corrigenda to 'Estimation of Stature from Long Limb Bones of American Whites and Negroes'. *American Journal of Physical Anthropology* **77: 355–56**.

FORENSIC MEDICINE AND PATHOLOGY

Brogdon, B.G. 1998. *Forensic Radiology*. Boca Raton, IL: CRC Press.

Byard, R.W. and Cohle, S.D. 1994. *Sudden Death in Infancy, Childhood and Adolescence*. Cambridge, Cambridge University Press.

Di Maio, V.J.M. 1999. *Gunshot Wounds*, 2nd edition. Boca Raton, IL: CRC Press.

Mason, J.K. 1989. *Paediatric Forensic Medicine and Pathology*. London: Chapman & Hall Medical.

Mason, J.K. and Perdue, B.N. 1999. *The Pathology of Trauma*, 3rd edition. London: Arnold.

McClay, W. 1996. *Clinical Forensic Medicine*. London: Greenwich Medical Media.

Robinson, S. 1996. *Principles of Forensic Medicine*. London: Greenwich Medical Media.

Saukko, P. and Knight, B. 2003. *Knight's Forensic Pathology*, 3rd edition. London: Arnold.

Stark, M.M. (ed.) 2000. *A Physicians' Guide to Clinical Forensic Medicine*. Totowa, NJ: Humana Press.

Valdés-Dapena, M. 1993. *Histopatholgy Atlas for Sudden Infant Death Syndrome*. Washington, DC: AFIP.

Whittaker, D. and MacDonald, D. 1989. *A Colour Atlas of Forensic Dentistry*. London: Wolfe Medical Publications.

MEDICAL ETHICS

BMA 2001. *The Medical Profession and Human Rights: A Handbook for a Changing Agenda*. London: BMA.

Mason, J. and McCall, R. 1999. *Law and Medical Ethics*. London: Butterworth Tolley.

Palls, C. and Harley, D.H. 1996. *ABC of Brainstem Death*, 2nd edition. London: BMJ Books.

TOXICOLOGY

Ellenhorn, M.J. 1997. *Ellenhorn's Medical Toxicology*, 2nd edition. Baltimore, MD: Williams and Wilkins.

WEBSITES

Amnesty International	www.amnesty.org.uk
British Medical Association	www.bma.org.uk
International Red Cross	www.ifr.org
Physicians for Human Rights	www.phsusa.org
United Nations	www.un.org
World Medical Association	www.wma.net

Index

Note: Page numbers in *italic* indicate figures; **bold type** refers to tables